ANNALS OF
THE NEW YORK ACADEMY
OF SCIENCES

Volume 970

EDITORIAL STAFF

Executive Editor
BARBARA M. GOLDMAN

Managing Editor
JUSTINE CULLINAN

The New York Academy of Sciences
2 East 63rd Street
New York, New York 10021

THE NEW YORK ACADEMY OF SCIENCES
(Founded in 1817)

BOARD OF GOVERNORS, September 2001 – September 2002

TORSTEN N. WIESEL, *Chairman of the Board*
JOHN F. NIBLACK, *Vice Chairman of the Board*
BILL GREEN, *Past Chairman*

Honorary Life Governors
WILLIAM T. GOLDEN JOSHUA LEDERBERG
JOHN T. MORGAN, *Treasurer*

Governors

ELEANOR BAUM	D. ALLAN BROMLEY	KAREN E. BURKE
	LAWRENCE B. BUTTENWIESER PRAVEEN CHAUDHARI	
JOHN H. GIBBONS	MICHAEL GOLDEN	RONALD L. GRAHAM
JACQUELINE LEO	SANDRA PANEM	RICHARD A. RIFKIND
JOHN J. ROCHE		SARA LEE SCHUPF
JAMES H. SIMONS		LEE VANCE

HELENE L. KAPLAN, *Counsel* [ex officio]

ENDOCRINE HYPERTENSION

ANNALS OF THE NEW YORK ACADEMY OF SCIENCES
Volume 970

ENDOCRINE HYPERTENSION

Edited by Karel Pacak and Graeme Eisenhofer

The New York Academy of Sciences
New York, New York
2002

Copyright © 2002 by the New York Academy of Sciences. All rights reserved. Under the provisions of the United States Copyright Act of 1976, individual readers of the Annals *are permitted to make fair use of the material in them for teaching or research. Permission is granted to quote from the* Annals *provided that the customary acknowledgment is made of the source. Material in the* Annals *may be republished only by permission of the Academy. Address inquiries to the Permissions Department (permissions@nyas.org) at the New York Academy of Sciences.*

Copying fees: For each copy of an article made beyond the free copying permitted under Section 107 or 108 of the 1976 Copyright Act, a fee should be paid through the Copyright Clearance Center, Inc., 222 Rosewood Drive, Danvers, MA 01923 (www.copyright.com).

♾ *The paper used in this publication meets the minimum requirements of the American National Standard for Information Sciences—Permanence of Paper for Printed Library Materials, ANSI Z39.48-1984.*

Library of Congress Cataloging-in-Publication Data

International Workshop on Endocrine Hypertension (1st: 2001 : Bethesda, Md.)
   Endocrine hypertension / edited by Karel Pacak and Graeme Eisenhofer.
     p. cm. — (Annals of the New York Academy of Sciences ; v. 970)
   "This volume is the result of a workshop entitled First International Workshop on Endocrine Hypertension sponsored by the Pediatric and Reproductive Endocrinology Branch, National Institute of Child Health and Human Development, and the Office of Rare Diseases, National Institutes of Health held on November 16, 2001 in Bethesda, Maryland" — Contents p.
   Includes bibliographical references and indexes.
   ISBN 1-57331-418-8 (hardcover : alk. paper) . — ISBN 1-57331-419-6 (paper : alk. paper)
   1. Hypertension — Endocrine aspects — Congresses. 2. Pheochromocytoma — Complications — Congresses. 3. Adrenal glands — Diseases — Complications — Congresses.
   [DNLM: 1. Adrenal Gland Neoplasms — Congresses. 2. Pheochromocytoma — Congresses. 3. Cushing Syndrome — Congresses. 4. Hypertension — etiology — Congresses. WK 780 161e 2002]
I. Pacak, Karel. II. Eisenhofer, Graeme. III. Title. IV. Series.
   Q11 .N5 vol 970
   [RC685.H8]
   616.1'32—dc21

2002012378

GYAT/B-MP
Printed in the United States of America
ISBN 1-57331-418-8 (cloth)
ISBN 1-57331-419-6 (paper)
ISSN 0077-8923

ANNALS OF THE NEW YORK ACADEMY OF SCIENCES
Volume 970
September 2002

ENDOCRINE HYPERTENSION

Editors
KAREL PACAK AND GRAEME EISENHOFER

This volume is the result of the **First International Workshop on Endocrine Hypertension** presented by the Pediatric and Reproductive Endocrinology Branch, National Institute of Child Health and Human Development and the Office of Rare Diseases, National Institutes of Health, and held on November 16, 2001 in Bethesda, Maryland.

CONTENTS

Preface. *By* KAREL PACAK AND GRAEME EISENHOFER vii

Part 1. Pheochromocytoma

Pheochromocytoma: An Approach to Antihypertensive Management. *By* EMMANUEL L. BRAVO 1

New Insights into the Genetics of Familial Chromaffin Cell Tumors. *By* CHRISTIAN A. KOCH, ALEXANDER O. VORTMEYER, ZHENGPING ZHUANG, FREDERIEKE M. BROUWERS, AND KAREL PACAK 11

New Advances in the Biochemical Diagnosis of Pheochromocytoma: Moving beyond Catecholamines. *By* JACQUES W.M. LENDERS, KAREL PACAK, AND GRAEME EISENHOFER 29

New Therapeutic and Surgical Approaches for Sporadic and Hereditary Pheochromocytoma. *By* MCCLELLAN M. WALTHER 41

Radiopharmaceutical Treatment of Pheochromocytomas. *By* JAMES C. SISSON 54

Part 2. Hyperaldosteronism/Mineralocorticoid Excess

Primary Aldosteronism: Management Issues. *By* WILLIAM F. YOUNG, JR. 61

New Genetic Insights in Familial Hyperaldosteronism. *By* RICHARD V. JACKSON, ANTHONY LAFFERTY, DAVID J. TORPY, AND CONSTANTINE STRATAKIS 77

The Pathophysiology of Aldosterone in the Cardiovascular System. *By* RICARDO ROCHA AND JOHN W. FUNDER 89

Part 3. Cushing's Syndrome

Familial/Sporadic Glucocorticoid Resistance Syndrome and Hypertension. *By* TOMOSHIGE KINO, ALESSANDRA VOTTERO, EVANGELIA CHARMANDARI, AND GEORGE P. CHROUSOS 101

Diagnostic Tests for Cushing's Syndrome. *By* LYNNETTE K. NIEMAN 112

The Medical Management of Cushing's Syndrome. *By* DAMIAN MORRIS AND ASHLEY GROSSMAN 119

Association of Hypertension and Hypokalemia with Cushing's Syndrome Caused by Ectopic ACTH Secretion: A Series of 58 Cases. *By* DAVID J. TORPY, NANCY MULLEN, IOANNIS ILIAS, AND LYNNETTE K. NIEMAN 134

Part 4. Endocrine Hypertension in Children

Hypertension in Congenital Adrenal Hyperplasia and Apparent Mineralocorticoid Excess. *By* MARIA I. NEW 145

The Diagnosis and Management of Endocrine Tumors Causing Hypertension in Children. *By* KURT D. NEWMAN AND TODD PONSKY 155

Part 5. Novel Methods of Localization and Treatment of Endocrine Tumors Causing Hypertension

The Role of PET in Localization of Neuroendocrine and Adrenocortical Tumors. *By* BARBRO ERIKSSON, MATS BERGSTRÖM, ANDERS SUNDIN, CLAES JUHLIN, HÅKAN ÖRLEFORS, KJELL ÖBERG, AND BENGT LÅNGSTRÖM 159

Diagnostic Localization of Pheochromocytoma: The Coming of Age of Positron Emission Tomography. *By* KAREL PACAK, GRAEME EISENHOFER, JORGE A. CARRASQUILLO, CLARA C. CHEN, MILLIE WHATLEY, AND DAVID S. GOLDSTEIN 170

Genomic Medicine: Exploring the Basis of a New Approach to Endocrine Hypertension. *By* SALVATORE ALESCI, GEORGE P. CHROUSOS, AND KAREL PACAK 177

Index of Contributors 193

Financial assistance was received from:

- **OFFICE OF RARE DISEASES, NIH**
- **NATIONAL INSTITUTE OF CHILD HEALTH AND HUMAN DEVELOPMENT, NIH**

> The New York Academy of Sciences believes it has a responsibility to provide an open forum for discussion of scientific questions. The positions taken by the participants in the reported conferences are their own and not necessarily those of the Academy. The Academy has no intent to influence legislation by providing such forums.

Preface

KAREL PACAK[a] AND GRAEME EISENHOFER[b]

National Institute of Child Health and Human Development, and National Institute of Neurological Disorders and Stroke, National Institutes of Health, Bethesda, Maryland 20817, USA

Hypertension is a major risk factor for stroke, ischemic heart disease, cardiac failure, and other cardiovascular disorders. An endocrine etiology such as glucocorticoid or catecholamine excess or hyperaldosteronism is responsible for a relatively small proportion of cases of hypertension. The importance of endocrine hypertension, however, is that in most cases the cause is clear and can be traced to the actions of a hormone, often produced in excess by a tumor. That means that the condition and any accompanying cardiovascular sequelae are not only treatable, but also are usually curable by surgical removal of the source of excess hormone secretion. Where excess hormone action is not due to a distinct resectable source, the resulting hypertension is also usually easily treated, provided the underlying condition is identified.

The key for a clinician who encounters a patient with endocrine hypertension is to think of it and recognize it. This and subsequent good detective work is usually rewarded by a cured and grateful patient. The further good news is that advances in medical diagnostics, genetics, and recognition of familial forms of endocrine hypertension are making the detective work a lot easier. As a consequence, endocrine causes of hypertension are fast becoming more readily recognized among the general hypertensive population, with subsequent improved treatment outcomes.

The material in this volume was compiled from the proceedings of the First International Workshop on Endocrine Hypertension, which was held in Bethesda, Maryland on November 16, 2002. The emphasis of the workshop was on clinical implications of recent discoveries in the field of endocrine hypertension, with a focus on advances in genetics and diagnostics that have led to improved identification of endocrine causes of hypertension and methods for management or treatment of endocrine hypertension. The workshop featured

Address for correspondence: Dr. Karel Pacak, Chief, Unit on Clinical Neuroendocrinology, PREB, NICHD, NIH, Building 10, Room 9D42, 10 Center Drive, Bethesda, MD 20817-1583. Voice: 301-402-4594; fax: 301-402-4712.
karel@mail.nih.gov

presentations from a diverse range of internationally recognized leaders in the field of endocrine hypertension. Many attendees traveled to the one-day workshop from several different and distant countries. We are grateful for the time and effort of those who participated in the meeting and for the final contributions of the speakers to this volume. We are also grateful to the National Institute of Child Health and Human Develpment and the Office of Rare Diseases at the National Institutes of Health for sponsoring the workshop.

Pheochromocytoma

An Approach to Antihypertensive Management

EMMANUEL L. BRAVO

Cleveland Clinic Foundation, Cleveland, Ohio 44195, USA

ABSTRACT: Pheochromocytoma and paragangliomas are rare tumors of chromaffin tissue that secrete catecholamines either intermittently or continuously, producing hypertension with a constellation of symptoms and signs that can be frightening to the patient and that continue to provide perplexing problems for clinicians. With surgical treatment, symptoms will be relieved and hypertension normalized or ameliorated for patients who do not have malignant tumors. Appropriate antihypertensive drugs are used to manage hypertension, to control associated cardiovascular symptoms, and to prepare patients for operation. The question debated most often regarding medical therapy of pheochromocytoma is whether antihypertensive treatment regimens other than nonspecific alpha-blockade are just as effective and safe. Understanding the pathophysiologic mechanisms that sustain the hypertension and the pharmacology of antihypertensive agents allows better selection of antihypertensive therapy.

KEYWORDS: pheochromocytoma; high plasma catecholamine levels; hypertension; antihypertensive agents; sympathetic nervous system; neuropeptide Y (NPY) levels

PATHOPHYSIOLOGY

Neurohumoral Mechanisms

The hypertension that accompanies pheochromocytoma has generally been ascribed solely to the action of excessive circulating catecholamines on cardiovascular adrenergic receptors. Under these conditions, the activity of the sympathetic nervous system (SNS) is thought to be decreased reflexly or normal because of baroreceptor resetting, and neuronally released norepinephrine (NE) is thought to be of minor physiologic import in comparison to the effects of elevated circulating catecholamines. However, recent studies

---

Address for correspondence: Emmanuel L. Bravo, M.D., Cleveland Clinic Foundation, 9500 Euclid Avenue, Desk A51, Cleveland, OH 44195. Voice: 216-444-5980; fax: 216-444-9378.
bronofs@ccf.org

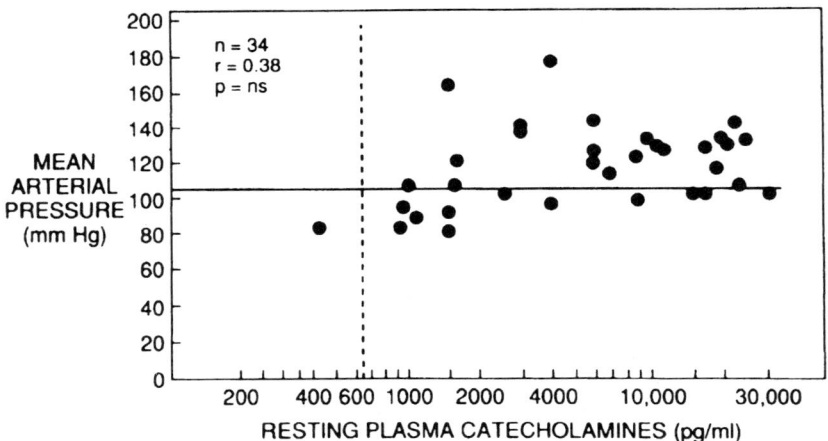

FIGURE 1. Relationship between the height of arterial pressure and circulating catecholamine (norepinephrine + epinephrine) levels in pheochromocytoma. (From Bravo et al.[2] Reprinted by permission.)

suggested that the SNS may play a role in blood pressure regulation in pheochromocytoma.[1] In patients with pheochromocytoma, blood pressure does not correlate with circulating catecholamines (FIG. 1).[2] In fact, some patients may have long periods of normotension despite high circulating catecholamines and paroxysms of hypertension without significant increases in plasma catecholamines (FIG. 2). Several studies demonstrate that under conditions of increased circulating catecholamines the SNS activity is either unchanged or enhanced and that SNS function is integral to the maintenance of the elevated blood pressure. *First*, 60-degree head-up tilt produces appropriate increases in heart rate and increases or unchanged diastolic blood pressure,[3] indicating intact baroreflex arc. *Second*, the oral administration of clonidine (a centrally acting antihypertensive agent that inhibits neurally mediated catecholamine release) rapidly decreases blood pressure and heart rate, but has no effect on plasma catecholamines (FIG. 3).[4] This indicates that biologically effective release of norepinephrine from axon terminals is maintained in pheochromocytoma and could contribute to the hypertension. *Third*, Johnson and coworkers[5] demonstrated that blood pressure during catecholamine infusions in rats is dependent upon a paradoxical increase in the activity of the SNS. This paradoxical increase in neuronal norepinephrine release appears to be the result of three factors: loading of sympathetic terminals with catecholamines, increased neuronal impulse frequency, and desensitization of prejunctional $alpha_2$ adrenergic receptors located in the noradrenergic terminal, which leads to enhanced release of neurotransmitter during nerve stimulation.[6] *Fourth*, Tsujimoto and coworkers[7] reported that

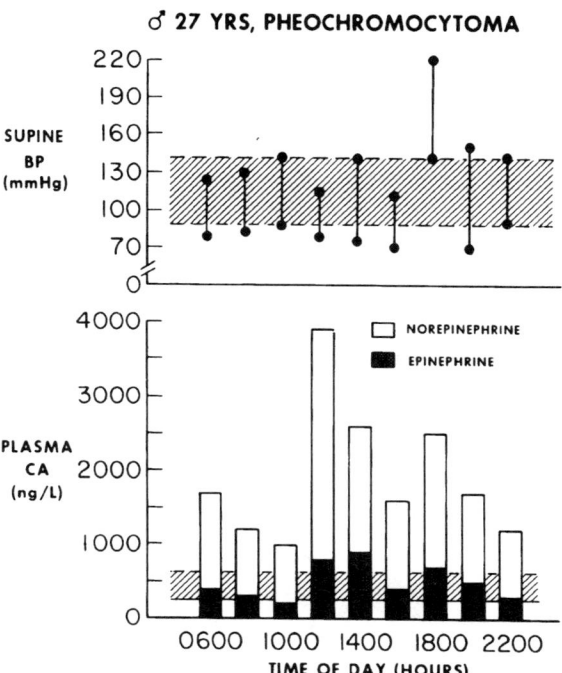

FIGURE 2. Plasma catecholamine concentrations and simultaneously recorded arterial blood pressure in a patient with adrenal pheochromocytoma. Each blood pressure point shown is the average of at least three determinations taken one minute apart. The cross-hatched area defines the upper limits for systolic blood pressure (140 mmHg) and diastolic blood pressure (90 mmHg). For plasma catecholamines, the cross-hatched area represents the mean (260 pg/ml) and +2 SD (580 pg/ml) of values obtained in 26 normotensive patients. All measurements were taken in the fasting state, after 30 minutes' supine rest, at 2-hour intervals from 6:00 AM to 10:00 PM.

elimination of sympathetic nerve activity by pithing caused a greater reduction of blood pressure in pheochromocytoma-bearing rats than in age-matched, unimplanted rats. Additionally, Prokocimer and coworkers found that both clonidine and chlorisondamine, a ganglion blocker, markedly decreased blood pressure in intact rats with pheochromocytoma.[8] However, the observation that the blood pressure in pithed pheochromocytoma rats is further reduced by phentolamine, an alpha-adrenergic antagonist, suggests that high concentrations of circulating catecholamines are also involved in the maintenance of elevated blood pressure.

Neuropeptide Y (NPY) values are increased in plasma and tumors of patients with pheochromocytoma (FIG. 4).[9-13] The peptide causes direct vasoconstriction, especially of small arterioles, and also potentiates NE-induced vasoconstriction.[14,15] NPY exerts its effect by interacting with vascular G-

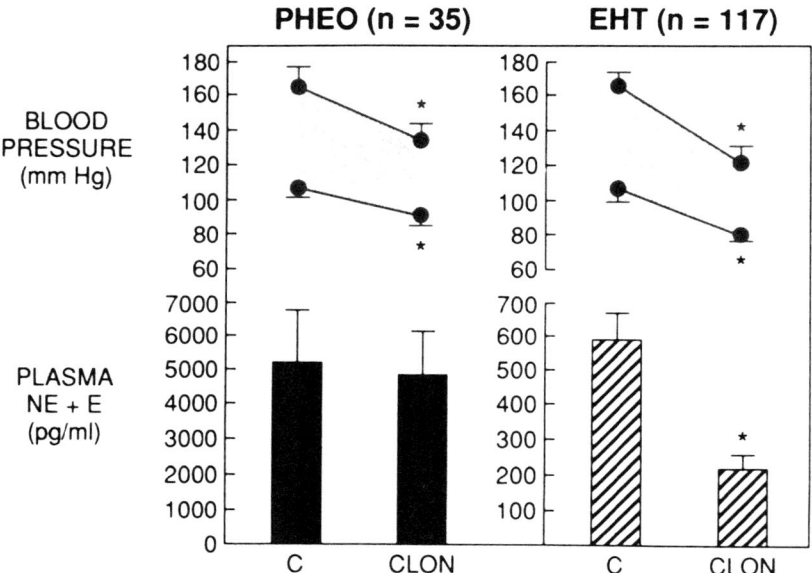

FIGURE 3. Blood pressure and plasma catecholamine responses to oral clonidine in patients with pheochromocytoma and essential hypertension. C = control; Clon = 3 hours after a single oral dose (0.3 mg) of clonidine. (From Bravo and Gifford.[31] Reprinted by permission.)

protein–coupled NPY receptors, which results in the mobilization of intracellular calcium and inhibition of adenylate cyclase.[16,17] This action is independent of alpha-adrenergic mechanisms. Indeed, Lunberg and coworkers have reported that preoperative alpha-blockade with 200 mg of phenoxybenzamine daily did not prevent the hypertensive response induced by surgical manipulation of an adrenal pheochromocytoma when both plasma NE and NPY levels were markedly increased.[12] These studies indicate that NPY released from pheochromocytoma may be partly responsible for some of the cardiovascular symptoms of these patients. Further, they suggest that alpha-adrenergic blockade may not be effective in decreasing arterial blood pressure when NPY is concomitantly released by a pheochromocytoma.

Hemodynamic Characteristics

Systemic administration of norepinephrine plus epinephrine increases cardiac rate and systemic vascular resistance, enhances cardiac contractility, and decreases venous compliance. From these findings the concept has developed that pheochromocytoma is a hyperkinetic, vasoconstrictive, hypovolemic form of hypertension. While it is clear that the hypertensive crisis of pheo-

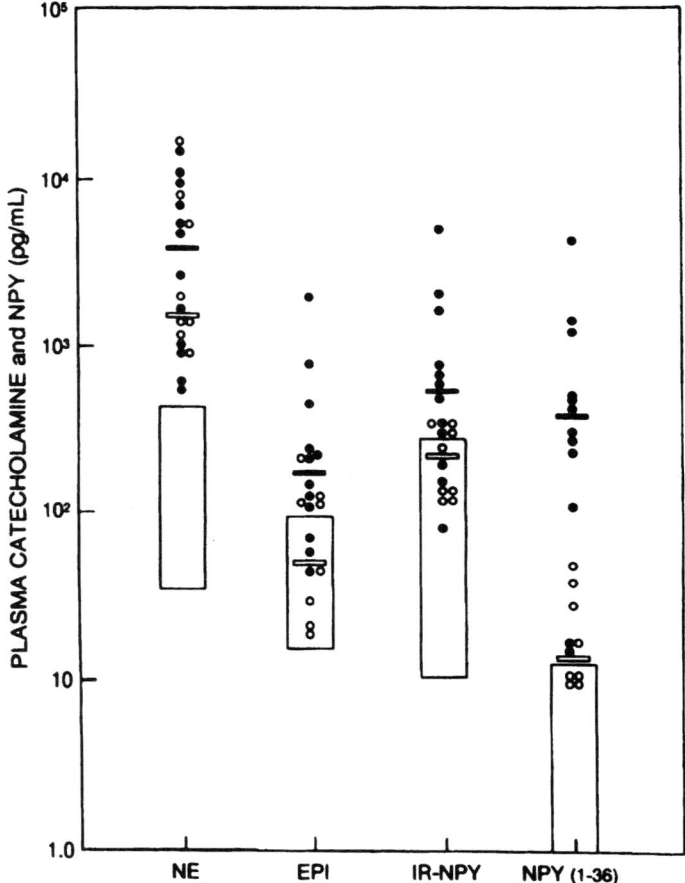

FIGURE 4. Levels of plasma norepinephrine (NE), epinephrine (EPI), immunoreactive neuropeptide Y (IR-NPY), and NPY (1-36) (determined by RIA coupled to reverse phase-HPLC) in patients with an adrenal (*solid circle*) or extraadrenal (*open circle*) pheochromocytoma. The rectangles in each lane indicate the normal range. (NE 126–402, 218; EPI 24–78, 42; IR-NPY 10–271, 174; NPY (1–36) <10–12, 10; range and median for the respective peptides). The median for each group is indicated by the transverse bars (*solid bar:* adrenal pheochromocytomas; *hollow bar:* extraadrenal pheochromocytomas).

chromocytoma mimics the hemodynamic responses to acute administration of catecholamines, we found[3] that under steady-state periods, despite having 10-fold higher levels of circulating catecholamines, pheochromocytoma patients have hemodynamic characteristics similar to patients with essential hypertension and that increased total peripheral resistance was primarily responsible for the maintenance of hypertension.

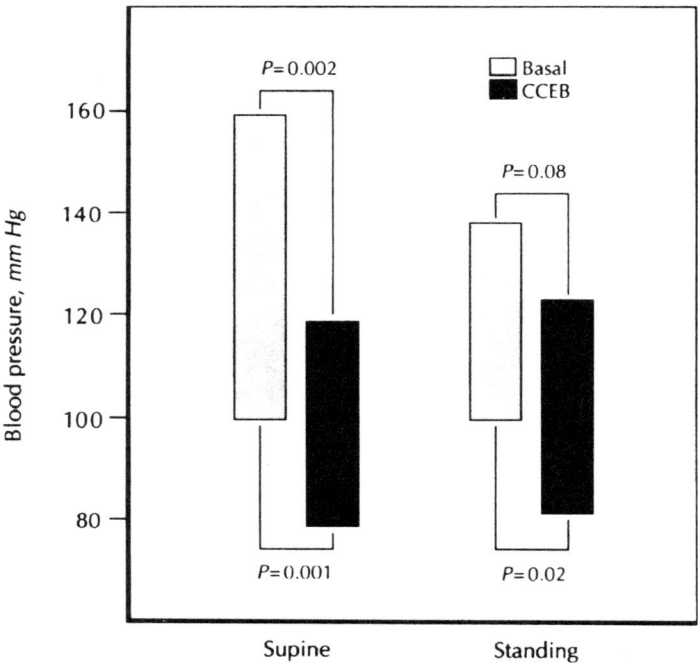

FIGURE 5. Blood pressure response to calcium antagonists in pheochromocytoma. Bars represent the mean systolic and diastolic blood pressures from 10 patients with surgically diagnosed pheochromocytoma. Patients received either verapamil-SR (120 to 240 mg daily; $n = 5$) or nifedipine-XL (30 to 90 mg daily; $n = 5$) for 6 to 8 weeks. The blood pressure values reported here were obtained immediately before drug administration and before the surgical procedure. Calcium antagonists maintained blood pressure at normal levels, and patients were symptom-free throughout the study period. Before drug treatment, patients had reduction in systolic blood pressure with standing. This reduction was completely eliminated during treatment. (From Bravo.[27] Reprinted by permission.)

ANTIHYPERTENSIVE AGENTS USED IN THE MANAGEMENT OF PHEOCHROMOCYTOMA

Nonselective Alpha-Adrenergic Blocker

Phenoxybenzamine (POB) hydrochloride has long been considered the drug of choice to control blood pressure and prevent symptomatic paroxysms. The theoretical advantages of POB relate to its ability to permit intravascular volume expansion and to block alpha-adrenergic receptors noncompetitively, which makes it difficult for released catecholamines to overcome its blocking effect.[18] The disadvantages are many. *First*, expansion of intravascular volume with alpha-adrenergic blocking agents takes 2 to 3 weeks. Hypovolemia can be corrected much more expeditiously by administering two to three units of whole blood or other volume expanders within 12 hours preoperatively. *Second,* despite adequate alpha-blockade, total elimination of cardiovascular disturbance is seldom achieved, and significant elevations of blood pressure are to be anticipated during manipulation of the tumor. Blunted maximal response to catecholamines may not be as persistent because of so-called spare alpha receptors in vascular smooth muscle.[19] Further, there may be concomitant release of NPY, which has direct vasoconstrictive effects independent of alpha-adrenergic receptor mechanisms. *Third,* alpha-blockade that is too vigorous and prolonged contributes to the hypotensive state that follows removal of the tumor. Since the drug inactivates alpha-adrenergic receptors irreversibly, the duration of its effect is dependent not only on the presence of the drug, but also on the rate of synthesis of alpha-adrenergic receptors. *Fourth,* it produces significant orthostatic hypotension and reflex tachycardia. The latter results from enhanced release of NE (because of the alpha$_2$-blockade) and decreased inactivation of the amine because of inhibition of neuronal and extraneuronal uptake mechanisms. *Finally,* there is no evidence that alpha-blockade has reduced perioperative mortality. In 63 consecutive patients with pheochromocytoma treated at the Cleveland Clinic, Boutros and coworkers[20] reported similar perioperative results whether or not patients received preoperative alpha-blockade.

Selective Alpha$_1$-Receptor Antagonists

Prazosin, terazosin, and doxazosin have been used to circumvent some of the disadvantages of POB. Because they do not block presynaptic alpha$_2$ receptors, this class of drugs does not enhance NE release and therefore does not produce reflex tachycardia.[21] They also have a shorter duration of action permitting more rapid adjustment of dosage and decreasing the duration of postoperative hypotension.

Calcium Channel Antagonists

All calcium channel antagonists lower blood pressure by relaxing arteriolar smooth muscle and decreasing peripheral vascular resistance. They exert their antihypertensive effect by inhibiting NE-mediated release of intracellular calcium and/or transmembrane calcium influx in vascular smooth muscle.[22] Thus, these agents have been shown to control blood pressure in pheochromocytoma.[23–26] These agents have the advantage of not producing overshoot hypotension or orthostatic hypotension and therefore may be used safely in patients who are normotensive but have occasional episodes of paroxysmal hypertension. Calcium channel antagonists are useful in managing patients with cardiovascular complications because they prevent catecholamine-induced coronary vasospasm and myocarditis. In doses of 30 to 90 mg/day, nifedipine gastrointestinal transport system (GITS) normalizes blood pressure in hypertensive patients and prevents the hypertensive response to provocative challenge (FIG. 4).[27] Nicardipine hydrochloride has been given as continuous intravenous infusion during surgery to control paroxysmal rises in blood pressure during tumor manipulations.[28] In more resistant cases, calcium channel antagonists can be combined with specific alpha$_1$-receptor antagonists with successful control of blood pressure and associated symptoms.

Beta-Blocking Agents

Beta-blocking agents are contraindicated in the absence of alpha-blockade because alpha$_1$ vasoconstriction mediated by high levels of circulating catecholamines would then be unopposed by the vasodilating beta$_2$ receptors, leading to exacerbation of hypertension and pulmonary edema, perhaps due to the negative isotropic effect of the beta-blockade. The alpha- and beta-blocking drug labetalol has been effective both orally and intravenously in controlling the hypertension of pheochromocytoma although the beta-blocking properties predominate.[29] Paradoxical hypertensive responses have been reported with this drug.[30]

Centrally Acting Alpha$_2$-Agonist

Clonidine has been shown to reduce blood pressure in patients with pheochromocytoma just as much as it does in patients with primary hypertension during clonidine suppression tests.[4] However, clonidine has not been used extensively in the preoperative management of pheochromocytoma because of the potential for rebound hypertension.

SUMMARY

The hypertension in pheochromocytoma is a complex process influenced by both the sympathetic nervous system and circulating catecholamines, as well as alterations in cardiovascular response, abnormalities in vascular smooth muscle calcium homeostasis, and perhaps increased release of NPY. The results of these studies provide a framework for a rational approach to hypertension therapy of this rare but intriguing endocrine-related hypertensive disorder. Appropriately used calcium channel antagonists and selective alpha$_1$-receptor blockers are effective and safe and have none of the adverse effects associated with nonspecific alpha-blockade.

REFERENCES

1. BRAVO, E.L., R.C. TARAZI, F.M. FOUAD, *et al*. 1982. Blood pressure regulation in pheochromocytoma. Hypertension **4** (Suppl II): 193–199.
2. BRAVO, E.L., R.C. TARAZI, R.W. GIFFORD, JR. & D.H. STEWART. 1979. Circulating and urinary catecholamines in pheochromocytoma: diagnostic and pathophysiologic implications. N. Engl. J. Med. **301**: 682–686.
3. BRAVO, E.L., F.M. FOUAD-TARAZI, G. ROSSI, *et al*. 1990. A reevaluation of the hemodynamics of pheochromocytoma. Hypertension **15**: I128–I131.
4. BRAVO, E.L., R.C. TARAZI, F.M. FOUAD, *et al*. 1981. Clonidine-suppression test: a useful aid in the diagnosis of pheochromocytoma. N. Engl. J. Med. **305**: 623–626.
5. JOHNSON, M.D., P.G. SMITH, E. MILLS & S.M. SCHANBERG. 1999. Paradoxical elevation of sympathetic activity during catecholamine infusion in rats. J. Pharmacol. Exp. Ther. **227**: 254–259.
6. LANGER, S.Z., I. CAVERO & R. MASSINGHAM. 1980. Recent developments in noradrenergic neurotransmission and its relevance to the mechanism of action of certain antihypertensive agents. Hypertension **2**: 372–382.
7. TSUJIMOTO, G., K. HONDA, B.B. HOFFMAN & K. HASHIMOTO. 1987. Desensitization of postjunctional alpha 1- and alpha 2-adrenergic receptor-mediated vasopressor responses in rat harboring pheochromocytoma. Circ. Res. **61**: 86–98.
8. PROKOCIMER, P.G., M. MAZE & B.B. HOFFMAN. 1987. Role of the sympathetic nervous system in the maintenance of hypertension in rats harboring pheochromocytoma. J. Pharmacol. Exp. Ther. **241**: 870–874.
9. DES SENANAYAKE, P., J. DENKER, E.L. BRAVO & R.M. GRAHAM. 1995. Production, characterization, and expression of neuropeptide Y by human pheochromocytoma. J. Clin. Invest. **96**: 2503–2509.
10. ADRIAN, T.E., J.M. ALLEN, G. TERENGHI, *et al*. 1983. Neuropeptide Y in phaeochromocytomas and ganglioneuroblastomas. Lancet **2**: 540–542.
11. CORDER, R., B. SHAPIRO, P.J. LOWRY, *et al*. 1986. Relationship between tumor and plasma concentrations of neuropeptide Y in patients with adrenal medullary phaeochromocytoma. J. Hypertens. **4**: S193–S195.
12. LUNDBERG, J.M., T. HOKFELT, A. HEMSEN, *et al*. 1986. Neuropeptide Y-like immunoreactivity in adrenaline cells of adrenal medulla and in tumors and plasma of pheochromocytoma patients. Regul. Pept. **13**: 169–182.
13. O'HARE, M.M. & T.W. SCHWARTZ. 1989. Expression and precursor processing of neuropeptide Y in human pheochromocytoma and neuroblastoma tumors. Cancer Res. **49**: 7010–7014.
14. WAHLESTEDT, C., L. EDVINSSON, E. EKBLAD & R. HAKANSON. 1985. Neuropeptide Y potentiates noradrenaline-evoked vasoconstriction: mode of action. J. Pharmacol. Exp. Ther. **234**: 735–741.
15. MACHO, P., R. PEREZ, J.P. HUIDOBRO-TORO & R.J. DOMENECH. 1989. Neuropeptide Y (NPY): a coronary vasoconstrictor and potentiator of catecholamine-induced coronary constriction. Eur. J. Pharmacol. **167**: 67–74.
16. LUNDBERG, J.M. & K. TATEMOTO. 1982. Pancreatic polypeptide family (APP, BPP, NPY and PYY) in relation to sympathetic vasoconstriction resistant to alpha-adrenoceptor blockade. Acta Physiol. Scand. **116**: 393–402.

17. HERZOG, H.Y., Y.J. HORT, H.J. BALL, et al. 1992. Cloned human neuropeptide Y receptor couples to two different second messenger systems. Proc. Natl. Acad. Sci. USA **89:** 5794–5798.
18. HAMILTON, C.A., J.L. REID & D.J. SUMNER. 1983. Acute effects of phenoxybenzamine on alpha-adrenoceptor responses in vivo and in vitro: relation of in vivo pressor responses to the number of specific adrenoceptor binding sites. J. Cardiovasc. Pharmacol. **5:** 868–873.
19. HAMILTON, C., H. DALRYMPLE & J. REID. 1982. Recovery in vivo and in vitro of alpha-adrenoceptor responses and radioligand binding after phenoxybenzamine. J. Cardiovasc. Pharmacol. 4(Suppl 1): S125–S128.
20. BOUTROS, A.R., E.L. BRAVO, G. ZANETTIN & R.A. STRAFFON. 1990. Perioperative management of 63 patients with pheochromocytoma. Cleveland Clin. J. Med. **57:** 613–617.
21. HOFFMAN, B.B. 2001. Catecholamines, sympathomimetic drugs, and adrenergic receptor antagonists. *In* Goodman & Gillman The Pharmacological Basis of Therapeutics, 10th ed., chapt. 10. J.G. Hardman & L.E. Lombard, Eds. :215–268. McGraw Hill. New York.
22. LEHMANN, H.U., H. HOCHREIN, E. WITT & H.W. MIES. 1983. Hemodynamic effects of calcium antagonists [review]. Hypertension **5:** II66–II73.
23. TAKAHASHI, S., T. NAKAI, R. FUJIWARA, et al. 1989. Effectiveness of long-acting nifedipine in pheochromocytoma. Jpn. Heart J. **30:** 751–757.
24. LENDERS, J.W., H.E. SLUITER, T. THIEN & J. WILLEMSEN. 1985. Treatment of a phaeochromocytoma of the urinary bladder with nifedipine. Br. Med. J. Clin. Res. **290:** 1624–1625.
25. PROYE, C., D. THEVENIN, P. CECAT, et al. 1989. Exclusive use of calcium channel blockers in preoperative and intraoperative control of pheochromocytomas: hemodynamics and free catecholamine assays in ten consecutive patients. Surgery **106:** 1149–1154.
26. FAVRE, L. & M.B. VALLOTTON. 1986. Nifedipine in pheochromocytoma [letter]. Ann. Intern. Med. **104:** 125.
27. BRAVO, E.L. 2001. Secondary hypertension: adrenal and nervous systems. *In* Hypertension: Mechanisms and Therapy. N.K. Hollenberg, Volume Ed. :118–143. Atlas of Heart Diseases, 3rd ed. E. Braunwald, Ed. Current Medicine. Philadelphia, PA.
28. TOKIOKA, H., T. TAKAHASHI, Y. KOSOGABE, et al. 1988. Use of nicardipine hydrochloride to control circulatory fluctuations during resection of a phaeochromocytoma. Br. J. Anaesth. **60:** 582–587.
29. NAVARATNARAJAH, M. & D.C. WHITE. 1984. Labetalol and phaeochromocytoma. Br. J. Anaesth. **56:** 1179.
30. BRIGGS, R.S.J., A.J. BIRTWELL & J.E.F. POHL. 1978. Hypertensive response to labetalol in phaeochromocytoma. Lancet **1:** 1045–1046.
31. BRAVO, E.L. & R.W. GIFFORD, JR. 1993. Pheochromocytoma. *In* Endocrine Crises. K.P. Ober, Ed. W.B. Saunders Co. Philadelphia, PA. [Endocrinol. Metab. Clin. N. Amer. **22:** 329–341.

New Insights into the Genetics of Familial Chromaffin Cell Tumors

CHRISTIAN A. KOCH,[a] ALEXANDER O. VORTMEYER,[b] ZHENGPING ZHUANG,[b] FREDERIEKE M. BROUWERS,[a] AND KAREL PACAK[a]

[a]*National Institute of Child Health and Human Development, Pediatric and Reproductive Endocrinology Branch, National Institutes of Health, Bethesda, Maryland 20892, USA*

[b]*Surgical Neurology Branch, NINDS, National Institutes of Health, Bethesda, Maryland 20892, USA*

ABSTRACT: We review genetic aspects and recent advances in our understanding of the molecular pathogenesis of familial chromaffin cell tumors (pheochromocytoma, paraganglioma). About 10 percent of pheochromocytomas are familial and occur as part of multiple endocrine neoplasia type 2 (MEN 2), von Hippel–Lindau (VHL) disease, and neurofibromatosis type 1 (NF 1). A subset of paragangliomas, tumors that can also produce and secrete catecholamines, are also familial and occur in patients with germline mutations in genes that encode subunits of the mitochondrial complex II. The precise molecular mechanisms underlying the pathogenesis of chromaffin cell tumors remain widely unknown, although recent studies in hereditary tumors help elucidate their development. In MEN 2, overrepresentation of mutant RET in selected adrenomedullary cells may be an important mechanism in initiating the formation of a pheochromocytoma. In VHL disease, pheochromocytoma development appears to occur according to Knudson's two-hit model, a *VHL* germline mutation and wildtype allelic deletion. Tumorigenesis of NF1-associated pheochromocytomas remains unknown, as does tumor formation (i.e., carotid body tumor) in patients with germline mutations in *SDHB*, *SDHC*, and *SDHD*, genes that encode subunits of the mitochondrial complex II, the smallest complex in the respiratory chain. Many genetic alterations have been found in sporadic chromaffin cell tumors. However, at present such genetic changes are difficult to place into context with regard to tumor formation and progression.

KEYWORDS: *RET*; *VHL*; *NF1*; *SDHD*; *SDHC*; *SDHB*; multiple endocrine neoplasia type 2; paraganglioma; pheochromocytoma; tumor formation; second hit

---

Address for correspondence: Christian A. Koch, M.D., FACP, Department of Medicine III, Endocrinology, Uniklinik, Phil.-Rosenthalstr. 27, 04103 Leipzig, Germany. Voice: 011 49 341 97 13 270; fax: 011 49 341 97 13 209.

Kochc@exchange.nih.gov

INTRODUCTION

Pheochromocytoma is a rare neural crest–derived neuroendocrine tumor composed of chromaffin tissue containing neurosecretory granules. The histologic term *chromaffin* stems from the observation that chromaffin tissue becomes dark after exposure to potassium dichromate. This characteristic chromaffin reaction depends on the formation of dark reaction products from the oxidation of catecholamines (mainly norepinephrine and epinephrine). In adults, most chromaffin cells are located in the adrenal medulla, but some are found in other tissues of the sympathetic nervous system, such as the organ of Zuckerkandl (between the aortic bifurcation and superior mesenteric artery). Many of the extra-adrenal chromaffin cells regress postnatally. In rare cases, this cell and tissue type gives rise to tumors, so-called paragangliomas.[1,2] Although paragangliomas may represent 15% of all chromaffin tissue–related tumors,[3] it is important to recall that there are also "nonchromaffin" paragangliomas (mainly the ones in the head and neck region). Such considerations are important not only for the diagnosis of these tumors (for instance, biochemically), but also when considering their pathogenesis. The classification of paragangliomas into chromaffin and nonchromaffin has limitations, since catecholamines have a very short half-life, and, therefore, fresh tissue must be rapidly put into the catecholamine-oxidizing potassium dichromate solution for a reliable statement regarding its "chromaffin" or "nonchromaffin" nature (nonchromaffin generally meaning containing no or little amounts of catecholamines such as norepinephrine and epinephrine). In spite of the wide acceptance to call paraganglia in the head and neck region such as the carotid bodies "nonchromaffin," suggesting that they do not contain any catecholamines, some investigators found dopamine and norepinephrine in carotid bodies.[4,5] The adrenal medulla has been regarded as the body's largest paraganglion.[2]

Approximately 90% of pheochromocytomas occur in the noninherited, sporadic form. The remainder represent inherited chromaffin cell tumors. At present, there are several major groups of familial "chromaffin" cell tumor syndromes, in which the respective inherited genetic defect has been identified: multiple endocrine neoplasia type 2 (MEN 2) caused by germline mutations in *RET*, von Hippel–Lindau (VHL) disease caused by germline mutations in *VHL*, neurofibromatosis type 1 (NF1) caused by germline mutations in *NF1*, and hereditary paraganglioma in patients with germline mutations in the SDHB, SDHC, or SDHD genes.[6–19]

In general, patients who are genetically predisposed to develop pheochromocytoma present at a younger age and usually have bilateral tumors compared to patients with sporadic pheochromocytoma.[20] Commercial testing for germline mutations in *RET, VHL*, and *SDHD, SDHC*, and *SDHB* now facilitates a more timely diagnosis of the underlying genetic syndrome. Genetic testing also helps reclassify patients with sporadic tumors, as 8% of patients with apparently sporadic pheochromocytomas prove to have germline mutations in *VHL*.[12,21,22] Seven percent of patients with apparently sporadic medullary thyroid carcinoma (usually the initial manifestation of MEN 2) turn out to have germline mutations in *RET*. Thus, it is considered justifiable to perform *RET* mutation analysis in all patients with medullary thyroid carcinoma.[23,24]

In the following, we discuss new genetic insights of familial "chromaffin" cell tumors by subdividing this heterogeneous group into the respective gene-related syndrome.

MULTIPLE ENDOCRINE NEOPLASIA TYPE 2 (MEN 2)

The most common organ affected in MEN 2 is the thyroid gland, which contains the so-called C (calcitonin-producing) cells. C cells are neural crest–derived as are chromaffin cells. All patients with MEN 2 develop medullary thyroid carcinoma and the majority of patients with MEN 2 have MEN 2A. MEN 2A was first described in 1961 by Sipple and is defined by the occurrence of medullary thyroid carcinoma, pheochromocytoma, and hyperparathyroidism caused by parathyroid gland hyperplasia/adenoma.[8,16,25] The prevalence of MEN 2 is similar to that of VHL disease with 1 in 35,000 individuals being affected. Kindreds with MEN 2 are found worldwide.[26] A rare variant of MEN 2A is familial medullary thyroid carcinoma associated with Hirschprung's disease,[27–29] an interesting combination in view of the molecular pathogenesis, as described below. There are also patients with Hirschsprung's disease alone who have germline mutations in *RET* (30%). MEN 2B represents about 5% of all MEN 2 cases and is defined by the presence of medullary thyroid carcinoma, pheochromocytoma, and associated abnormalities including mucosal neuromas (within the lips, the gastrointestinal tract, on the tongue tip and eyelids), abnormal corneal nerve fibers, and marfanoid habitus.[30] In contrast to patients with Marfan syndrome, however, patients with MEN 2B do not have lens or aortic abnormalities. Mucosal neuromas within the lips often give the lips a blubbery/bumpy look. Physical examination is remarkable for these associated abnormalities. For instance, slit lamp examination may reveal hypertrophied corneal nerves. Often, patients have an acromegaloid appearance. Intestinal ganglioneuromatosis may cause diarrhea alternating with constipation or even obstruction. Most reports state a (clinical) pheochromocytoma prevalence of approximately 50% in patients with MEN 2. This may represent an underestimation of the true prevalence of pheochromocytoma in patients with MEN 2. Whether all patients who have a germline mutation in *RET* develop a pheochromocytoma during their lifetime can only be determined by autopsy studies, since many tumors may remain clinically undiagnosed.

The gene responsible for MEN 2 is *RET*.[31] *In vitro* experiments indicate that *RET* is a proto-oncogene.[32] *RET* is specifically expressed in neural crest–derived cells, such as the calcitonin-producing C cells in the thyroid gland and the catecholamine-producing chromaffin cells in the adrenal gland. In patients with MEN 2A, hyperparathyroidism is reported to occur in approximately 20% of cases, whereas in patients with MEN 2B, hyperparathyroidism is uncommon or lacking, although both MEN 2A and MEN 2B are caused by germline mutations in *RET*. *RET* is located on chromosome 10q11.2 and encodes a receptor tyrosine kinase, RET protein, whose ligands are glial cell line–derived neurotrophic factor (GDNF), neurturin, artemin, and persephin, all structurally related to transforming growth factor (TGF)-beta.[33] *RET* activation by the GDNF family ligands appears to occur via a unique membrane-bound multicomponent receptor complex consisting of a glycosyl-phosphatidylinositol–anchored coreceptor (GFR alpha 1–4) as the ligand-binding domain and RET protein as the signaling component of the ligand–receptor complex.[9,34,35] The downstream signaling pathway of RET is complex and includes RAS/extracellular signal-regulated kinase (ERK).[33,36] This pathway has an impact on cell survival and proliferation. *RET* consists of 21 exons with 6 so-called hot-spot exons (exons 10, 11, 13, 14, 15, 16) in which mutations are identified in 97% of patients with MEN 2. *RET* germline mutation screening is commercially available and has widely replaced the cumbersome provocative testing of calcitonin stimulation (with calcium and/or pentagastrin). *RET* plays a role in normal gastrointestinal neuronal and kidney development as exemplified by the *RET* knockout mouse, which has a Hirschsprung-like phenotype and renal dys- or agenesis.[37,38] In patients with MEN 2, *RET* germline mutations are believed to be "activating." There are patients with Hirschsprung's disease and so-called "inactivating" *RET* germline mutations, and, moreover, patients with both MEN 2 and Hirschsprung's disease with germline mutations in codons 609, 618, and 620.[16]

A patient with known *RET* germline mutation may present with signs and symptoms suggestive of pheochromocytoma and positive biochemical tests as indicated by elevated plasma free metanephrines, but negative high-resolution imaging modalities such as magnetic resonance imaging and computed tomography, as well as ^{123}I- or ^{131}I- metaiodobenzylguanidine scanning. It presently remains unknown whether such a patient has a paraganglioma, pheochromocytoma, or adrenomedullary hyperplasia, which has been regarded as a precursor lesion for pheochromocytoma.[39,40] This scenario leads us to further ask why different, unrelated patients with MEN 2 and the same germline mutation in *RET* (for instance, TGC/GGC, codon 634) have a (biochemically and on imaging) diagnosable and treatable pheochromocytoma at different ages, some early in life (for instance, in the first decade), and others as late as in the 8th decade. This clinical observation suggests that a germline mutation in *RET* is obligatory but perhaps not suffi-

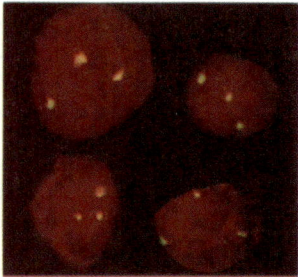 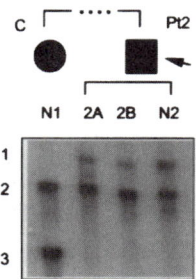

FIGURE 1. Duplication of mutant *RET* in trisomy 10 in MEN 2–related pheochromocytoma. Pheochromocytoma tumor cells are shown in red. The yellow signals are FISH markers for chromosome 10. Each tumor cell has trisomy 10. C, cousin; Pt2, patient; N, normal tissue; 2A and 2B, pheochromocytoma; 1–3 are alleles with allele 2 being the inherited, mutant *RET* allele shared by cousin C and patient Pt2. Modified from Huang/Koch et al.[42]

cient to cause tumor formation in MEN 2 *in vivo*. Other genetic hits may be required.

In analogy to another oncogene and receptor tyrosine kinase, *MET*, which has homology to *RET* and has recently been shown to cause tumorigenesis in patients with hereditary papillary renal carcinoma by imbalance between mutant and wild-type *MET* through trisomy 7,[41] we hypothesized that a similar mechanism may exist for *RET* in patients with MEN 2. In our study of MEN 2A–associated pheochromocytomas, we identified two possible mechanisms of tumorigenesis, both leading to overrepresentation of mutant *RET*: duplication of the mutant *RET* allele in trisomy 10 or loss of the wild-type allele[42] (FIG. 1). This finding of an allelic imbalance between the mutant and wild-type *RET* allele could be further confirmed in MEN 2A–related medullary thyroid carcinoma.[43] In addition, we could demonstrate overexpression of mutant *RET* by investigating the stable TT cell line, which is representative for MEN 2A–associated medullary thyroid carcinoma.[44,45] Similar findings of a second hit in an oncogene such as *RET* are reported by a recent study in another oncogene, *Kras2*.[46] *Ras* genes have been established as proto-oncogenes, but the dominant role of activated *ras* in cell transformation has been questioned. Zhang et al.[46] provided data (loss of wild-type *Kras2* with exclusive presence of mutant *Kras2* caused large lung tumors in mice), indicating that wild-type *Kras2* may have properties of a tumor suppressor gene and may be able to reduce the transforming potential of oncogenically activated *ras*.[47]

Considering these mechanisms of tumorigenesis, one might ask whether there are patients with MEN 2 and double mutations in *RET* which make both

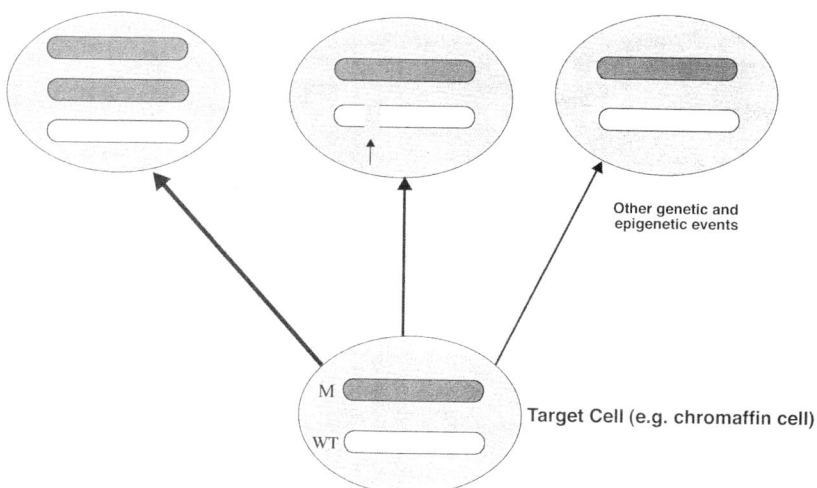

FIGURE 2. Proposed mechanisms of tumor formation in MEN 2. A target cell such as the adrenal chromaffin cell or the C-cell of the thyroid gland contains one mutant and one wild-type copy of *RET*. At some point during life, perhaps through replication errors of these dividing cells, selected cells in the target tissues acquire two mutant *RET* copies or lose the wild-type *RET* copy, which might trigger tumorigenesis.

alleles mutated. (In this case, after the additional somatic *RET* mutation at the wild-type allele, there would be no normal wild-type *RET* allele left in the tumor.) Indeed, there are reports on double or even multiple *RET* sequence alterations. However, the *RET* double mutation or sequence alteration occurred on the same allele, thus leaving the *RET* wild-type allele intact and balanced with the mutant allele.[48–51] The functional effect of such sequence alterations in *RET* remains to be determined. To our knowledge, there are no patients with MEN 2 and homozygous *RET* germline mutations.

On the other hand, not all MEN 2–associated tumors investigated by us revealed allelic imbalance between mutant and wild-type *RET*. In part, this may be related to the experimental analysis, for instance, the informative polymorphic markers used and whether microdissected or non-microdissected DNA had been analyzed.[43] More importantly, however, other mechanisms of tumor formation may have been responsible in these tumors (FIG. 2). Allele losses in MEN 2–associated pheochromocytomas have been reported to occur on 1p, 3p (including the VHL gene locus), 3q, and chromosome 22[7,52–56] (TABLE 1). The frequencies of such allele losses (in general above 50%) may even prove to be higher, when microdissection analysis is used.[57,58]

Since somatic mutations in *RET* and *VHL* are identified in a subset of sporadic pheochromocytomas (< 10% have mutations in *RET*, < 8% in

TABLE 1. Allele losses in MEN-2-associated pheochromocytoma

Chromosome	Frequency
1p	<100%
3p	<50%
3q	<60%
11p	<12%
17p	<12%
22	<60%

DATA SOURCE: Moley et al.[53]; Mulligan et al.[52]; Benn et al.[54]

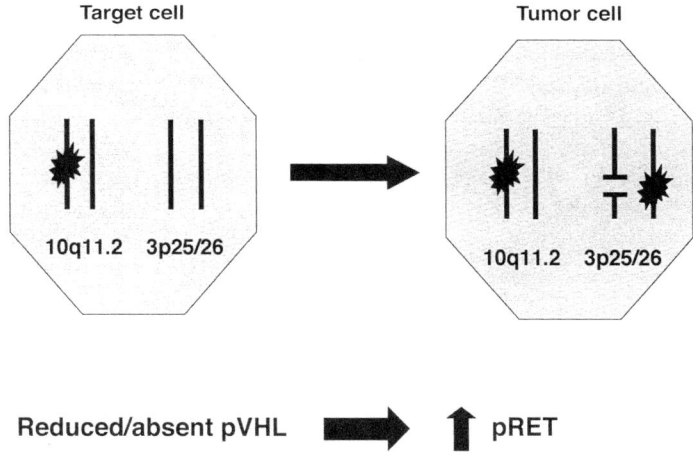

FIGURE 3. Model for somatic biallelic *VHL* inactivation in MEN 2 pheochromocytoma. Target cells such as the adrenal chromaffin cell or the C-cell of the thyroid gland contain one mutant and one wild-type copy of *RET*. Both *VHL* copies are intact. Upon inactivation of both *VHL* copies, tumor formation may occur, perhaps by accumulation of mutant RET.

VHL[7,21,59–68]), thereby suggesting a role in the pathogenesis of pheochromocytoma, we searched for a somatic biallelic inactivation of *VHL* in those MEN 2–associated pheochromocytomas that did not reveal allelic imbalance between mutant and wild-type *RET* alleles (FIG. 3). Somatic *VHL* gene deletion and mutation ("*VHL* knockout") could be identified in three of four MEN 2–related pheochromocytomas.[69] Absent or reduced VHL protein leads to decreased degradation of certain proteins which might include RET protein, thereby leading to accumulation of (mutant) RET protein.[70] Although these recent data are very helpful in better understanding the pathogenesis of MEN 2–related pheochromocytoma, further and more extensive studies are needed in delineating how these fascinating tumors develop.

PHEOCHROMOCYTOMA IN VON HIPPEL– LINDAU DISEASE TYPE 2

Von Hippel–Lindau disease is an autosomal dominantly inherited cancer syndrome in which affected individuals develop a variety of tumors including pheochromocytoma.[12,71] VHL disease is subdivided into VHL type 1 (without pheochromocytoma) and VHL type 2 (with pheochromocytoma). The prevalence of VHL disease is similar to that of MEN 2: affecting one in 35,000 individuals. Pheochromocytoma occurs in about 30% of patients with VHL disease and is the presenting manifestation in about 5% of cases.[12,72,73] As in other hereditary tumor syndromes, multifocal and bilateral tumors are expected, and are reported to occur (clinically) in 50% of patients. It is important to note that patients with VHL syndrome who undergo unilateral adrenalectomy for pheochromocytoma need lifelong follow-up to make timely diagnosis of another pheochromocytoma on the contralateral side or metastatic pheochromocytoma. Metastatic pheochromocytoma is more common in patients with VHL disease (about 25%) compared to patients with MEN 2 and neurofibromatosis type 1 (6%).[12,14,74]

The VHL tumor suppressor gene is ubiquitously expressed and located on chromosome 3p25-26. The cloned coding sequence comprises three exons. Most patients with VHL-associated pheochromocytoma have missense mutations.[22,75,76] There are genotype-specific VHL phenotypes. Germline mutations in the VHL gene have been catalogued (see http://www.ncifcrf.gov/research/kidney).[12,77] "Founder effects" may explain regional prevalence rates (e.g., the Black Forest area in Southern Germany, with the missense mutation tyrosine to histidine at codon 98 (Tyr98His) and subsequent high risk of pheochromocytoma).[74,78,79]

The VHL gene product forms a stable complex with the highly conserved transcription elongation factors that regulate RNA polymerase II elongation. Formation of this heterotrimeric complex with elongin B and C appears to be the tumor suppressor function of the VHL gene, since the majority of tumor-predisposing mutations of *VHL* disrupt the formation of this complex.[80,81] Normal VHL protein function leads to degradation of a proteasome complex.[70] Absent or reduced VHL protein may lead to accumulation of this proteasome complex, which may include proteins that are involved in cell proliferation.

According to Knudson's two-hit model, tumor formation in tumor suppressor gene-related neoplasms usually occurs by biallelic inactivation of the respective gene. In most cases, this includes a germline mutation and subsequent deletion of the wild-type allele. However, there are some patients with VHL type 1 disease (no pheochromocytoma) who do not have a *VHL* germline mutation. Instead, these patients have a *VHL* germline deletion, as discovered by fluorescence *in situ* hybridization of white blood cells, and *VHL* point mutation at the wild-type allele in the respective tumor.[82] More than 300 *VHL* germline mutations have been identified and 36 of them are associated with pheochromocytoma.[83,84] Most patients with VHL-associated pheochromocytoma have missense mutations.[22,75,76]

The "second hit" in VHL-associated pheochromocytomas could be shown as loss of heterozygosity at 3p25/26 in at least 93% of tumors.[7,56,85] The germline mutation/wild-type allelic deletion sequence in the VHL gene is found in renal carcinoma and in renal cysts of patients with VHL disease. Since renal cysts are benign structures, this might indicate that the "second hit" in these lesions occurs as an early developmental event.[86]

PHEOCHROMOCYTOMA IN NEUROFIBROMATOSIS TYPE 1

Neurofibromatosis type 1 (NF1) affects about one in 3000 individuals.[87] Pheochromocytoma is (clinically) diagnosed in fewer than 2% of such patients.[88] There are no autopsy studies on the true prevalence of pheochromocytoma in NF1, a disease inherited in an autosomal dominant manner.

Fewer than a quarter of NF1 patients with pheochromocytoma (that is, 0.25 from 2% = 0.5% of *all* patients with NF1) are diagnosed with bilateral pheochromocytomas, and fewer than 6% of pheochromocytomas in patients with NF1 are reportedly metastatic.[14]

The NF1 gene is a tumor-suppressor gene mapping to chromosome 17q11.2. It has a large gene size encompassing an open reading frame of 8454 nucleotides spanning approximately 300,000 nucleotides of genomic DNA. The mRNA comprises 12,000 nucleotides, and germline mutations in *NF1* range from nonsense and missense mutations to large deletions. The encoded protein is called neurofibromin and has similarity to a family of GTPase-activating proteins involved in downregulation of a cellular proto-oncogene, p21-*ras*. By affecting intrinsic GTP hydrolysis in the small G proteins, the RAS genes, signal transduction is controlled through these *RAS* pathways. *RAS* reportedly has a role in controlling cell growth and differentiation.[89]

Since *NF1* is a tumor-suppressor gene requiring biallelic inactivation for tumor formation according to Knudson's two-hit model, studies in this regard should demonstrate inactivation of both *NF1* copies via mutation, deletion, or other mechanisms. In mice heterozygous for one mutant *NF1* allele, 50% develop pheochromocytoma.[90] In patients with NF1-associated pheochromocytoma, loss of the wild-type *NF1* allele could be shown in three of seven tumors without knowing whether these patients had germline mutations in *NF1*.[91] In another study with six pheochromocytomas, none had neurofibromin expression, although neurofibromin is normally expressed in the adrenal gland. In addition, LOH could be shown in one of these six tumors without known *NF1* germline mutation.[92] Importantly, loss of neurofibromin can be seen in tumors from patients with and without NF.[87,93] Reduced or absent NF 1 gene expression was found in one of four sporadic adrenal pheochromocytomas.[93] Further work is required to elucidate the pathways of tumor development in NF1-associated pheochromocytoma.

HEREDITARY PARAGANGLIOMAS

Paragangliomas are neural crest–derived tumors arising in extra-adrenal chromaffin and nonchromaffin tissue. The estimated incidence of these tumors is one in 500,000 individuals.[94] The most common tumor site is the carotid body, a chemoreceptive organ that senses oxygen levels in the blood. In earlier reports, carotid bodies and other endocrine structures in the head and neck have been classified as paraganglia in the belief of a presumed neural connection with the sympathetic nervous system. Although the carotid bodies and other paraganglia in the head and neck are classified as "nonchromaffin," suggesting that they do not contain any catecholamines, some investigators found dopamine and norepinephrine in carotid bodies.[4,5] In this context it is important to recall that catecholamines have a very short half-life. Therefore, fresh tissue must be rapidly put into the catecholamine-oxidizing potassium dichromate solution for a reliable statement regarding its chromaffin or nonchromaffin nature (nonchromaffin generally meaning not containing catecholamines such as norepinephrine and epinephrine).

Fewer than a third of patients with paragangliomas have tumoral catecholamine excess, and fewer than 5% of carotid body paragangliomas have been shown to produce and secrete catecholamines.[95] Analogous to other tissue types such as the lung (small-cell lung cancer and ACTH or vasopressin production) or the uterine cervix (atypical carcinoid and ACTH or serotonin production), this underscores that the hormonal pattern (production and secretion) of the "same" tissue type can be different in mature and in less differentiated or "tumor" tissue.[96,97] Therefore, in contrast to normal nonchromaffin ("catecholamine-poor") paraganglia, paragangliomas arising from nonchromaffin paraganglia may produce and secrete hormones such as catecholamines, whereas paragangliomas arising from originally chromaffin ("catecholamine-rich") paraganglia may or may not.

At high altitudes or other conditions associated with chronic hypoxia, carotid bodies of humans may become hypertrophic and hyperplastic.[98–102] As in other (endocrine) organs, this does not necessarily represent the basis for tumorigenesis. For instance, adrenal hyperplasia after removal of the contralateral adrenal gland is temporary and does not necessarily lead to tumor formation.[1,2,103] Carotid body stimulation at high altitudes appears to be a temporary phenomenon, since hypoxia-adaptive mechanisms occur, such as increased production of red blood cells, which deliver oxygen to the tissues.

The genetic basis of paragangliomas remains largely unknown, although recent analyses of families with paraganglioma (approximately 40% are familial) revealed several possible susceptibility chromosomal loci for this tumor: PGL1 resulting from germline mutations in *SDHD* (the succinate-ubiquinone oxidoreductase subunit D gene) at 11q23, PGL2 mapping to 11q13 with a yet unidentified gene, PGL3 at 1q21 including the *SDHC* gene locus, and recently 1p36 including *SDHB*.[10,11,18,19,104,105] *SDHD*, *SDHC*, *SDHB*, and *SDHA* encode each a subunit of the mitochondrial respiratory chain complex II. This enzyme complex is important for the aerobic respiratory chain of eukaryotic cell mitochondria. The SDHD gene comprises three introns and four exons, *SDHC* consists of six exons, *SDHB* of eight exons, and *SDHA* of fifteen exons.[19]

Mutations in *SDHA* are not associated with hereditary paraganglioma, but with optic atrophy, ataxia, and myopathy. Heterozygous germline mutations in *SDHB* or *SDHC* have been identified in small subsets of patients with hereditary paragangliomas.[11,18] However, in these studies, there are only sparse data on LOH of the respective gene locus. In contrast, the majority of hereditary paragangliomas in patients with germline mutations in *SDHD* demonstrate LOH at 11q23, indicating a loss-of-function status which is commonly seen in tumor-suppressor gene-related disorders.[106,107] Of note, 11q23 contains many other genes besides *SDHD*.[10] Interestingly, sporadic adrenal pheochromocytomas may have somatic mutations in *SDHD*.[6] However, such somatic *SDHD* mutations occur in a low frequency (<10%) similar to the one seen with somatic *RET* and *VHL* mutations in sporadic pheochromocytomas (TABLE 2). It remains to be determined how paragangliomas develop by such mitochondrial complex II gene alterations.

As mentioned above, allele losses on chromosomes 1p, 3p, 3q, 17p, and 22q are common findings in familial and non-familial pheochromo-

TABLE 2. Frequency of mutations in *RET*, *VHL*, or *SDHD/C/B* in sporadic chromaffin cell tumors

Gene	Frequency
RET	<10%
VHL	<8%
SDHD	1/15
SDHC	0/24
SDHB	1/24

DATA SOURCES: Eng *et al.*[21]; Crossey *et al.*[68]; Hofstra *et al.*[60]; Rodien *et al.*,[111] 1997; Gimm *et al.*[6]; Astuti *et al.*[18]

cytomas, as indicated by comparative hybridization and microsatellite analyses.[7,52–56,108–110] Most of these allele losses are not clearly involved in tumorigenesis of pheochromocytomas. Accumulation of mutations and deletions in several genes in both familial and sporadic pheochromocytomas may develop during tumor progression. The specific role and function of these genes remains to be elucidated, that is, details of how mutations in different biochemical pathways might interact with each other to produce tumorigenesis. Future analyses of pheochromocytomas combining clinical and morphological observations with genetic investigations including microarray techniques, proteomics, and the yeast two-hybrid system may help answer these questions.

[Note added in proof: Recently, Neumann et al.[112] identified germline mutations in *Ret, VHL, SDHB*, or *SDHD* in up to 24% of 271 patients who presented with apparently sporadic pheochromocytoma.]

REFERENCES

1. LACK, E.E. 1994. Pathology of Adrenal and Extraadrenal Paraganglia. W.B. Saunders. Philadelphia, PA.
2. LACK, E.E. 1997. Tumors of the Adrenal and Extraadrenal Paraganglia. Armed Forces Institute of Pathology. Washington, DC.
3. WHALEN, R.K., A.F. ALTHAUSEN & G.H. DANIELS. 1992. Extraadrenal pheochromocytoma. J. Urol. **147:** 1–10.
4. LACK, E.E., A.R. PEREZ-ATAYDE & J.B. YOUNG. 1986. Carotid bodies in sudden infant death syndrome: a combined light microscopic, ultrastructural and biochemical study. Ped. Pathol. **6:** 335–350.
5. ZAPATA, P., A. HESS, E.L. BLISS, et al. 1969. Chemical, electron microscopic and physiological observations on the role of catecholamines in the carotid body. Brain Res. **14:** 473–496.
6. GIMM, O., M. ARMANIOS, H. DZIEMA, et al. 2000. Somatic and occult germline mutations in *SDHD*, a mitochondrial complex II gene, in nonfamilial pheochromocytoma. Cancer Res. **60:** 6822–6825.
7. BENDER, B.U., M. GUTSCHE, S. GLASKER, et al. 2000. Differential genetic alterations in von Hippel-Lindau syndrome-associated and sporadic pheochromocytomas. J. Clin. Endocrinol. Metab. **85:** 4568–4574.
8. HANSFORD, J.R. & L.M. MULLIGAN. 2000. Multiple endocrine neoplasia type 2 (MEN 2) and *RET*: from neoplasia to neurogenesis. J. Med. Genet. **37:** 817–827.
9. JHIANG, S.M. 2000. The RET protooncogene in human cancers. Oncogene **19:** 5590–5597.
10. BAYSAL, B.E., R.E FERRELL, J.E. WILLETT-BROZICK, et al. 2000. Mutations in *SDHD*, a mitochondrial complex II gene in hereditary paraganglioma. Science **287:** 848–851.
11. NIEMANN, S. & U. MULLER. 2000. Mutations in *SDHC* cause autosomal dominant paraganglioma type 3. Nat. Genet. **26:** 268–270.

12. WALTHER, M.M., R. REITER, H.R. KEISER, et al. 1999. Clinical and genetic characterization of pheochromocytoma in von Hippel-Lindau families: comparison with sporadic pheochromocytoma gives insight into natural history of pheochromocytoma. J. Urol. **162:** 659–664.
13. KORF, B.R. 2000. Malignancy in neurofibromatosis type 1. The Oncologist **5:** 477–485.
14. WALTHER, M.M., J. HERRING, E. ENQUIST, et al. 1999. Von Recklinghausen's disease and pheochromocytomas. J. Urol. **162:** 1582–1586.
15. PACAK, K., G.P. CHROUSOS, C.A. KOCH, et al. 2001. Pheochromocytoma: progress in diagnosis, therapy, and genetics. In Adrenal Disorders. A. Margioris & G.P. Chrousos, Eds. :379–413. Humana Press. New York.
16. ENG, C. 1999. RET protooncogene in the development of human cancer. J. Clin. Oncol. **17:** 380–393.
17. NILSSON, O., L.E. TISELL, S. JANSSON, et al. 1999. Adrenal and extraadrenal pheochromocytomas in a family with germline RET V804L mutation. JAMA **281:** 1587–1588.
18. ASTUTI, D., F. LATIF, A. DALLOL, et al. 2001. Gene mutations in the succinate dehydrogenase subunit SDHB cause susceptibility to familial pheochromocytoma and to familial paraganglioma. Am. J. Hum. Genet. **69:** 49–54.
19. BAYSAL, B., W.S. RUBINSTEIN & P.E.M. TASCHNER. 2001. Phenotypic dichotomy in mitochondrial complex II genetic disorders. J. Mol. Med. **79:** 495–503.
20. KOCH, C.A., D. MAURO, M.M. WALTHER, et al. 2002. Pheochromocytomas in VHL disease: distinct histopathologic phenotype compared to pheochromocytoma in multiple endocrine neoplasia type 2. Endocr. Pathol. **13:** 17–27.
21. ENG C., P.A. CROSSEY, L.M. MULLIGAN, et al. 1995. Mutations in the RET proto-oncogene and the von Hippel-Lindau disease tumor suppressor gene in sporadic and syndromic pheochromocytomas. J. Med. Genet. **32:** 934–937.
22. VAN DER HARST, E., R.R. DE KRIJGER, W.N. DINJENS, et al. 1998. Germline mutations in the VHL gene in patients presenting with pheochromocytoma. Int. J. Cancer **77:** 337–340.
23. WOHLK, N., G.J. COTE, M.M. BUGALHO, et al. 1996. Relevance of RET protooncogene mutations in sporadic medullary thyroid carcinoma. J. Clin. Endocrinol. Metab. **81:** 3740–3745.
24. DECKER, R.A., M.L. PEACOCK, M.J. BORST, et al. 1995. Progress in genetic screening of multiple endocrine neoplasia type 2A: is calcitonin obsolete? Surgery **118:** 257–263.
25. SIPPLE, J.H. 1961. The association of pheochromocytoma with carcinoma of the thyroid gland. Am. J. Med. **31:** 163–166.
26. GAGEL, R.F. 2001. Multiple endocrine neoplasia type 2. In DeGroot's Endocrinology, 4th ed. L. DeGroot & J.L. Jameson, Eds.: Vol. **3:** 2518–2532. W.B. Saunders. Philadelphia, PA.
27. ENG, C. 1996. Seminars in medicine of the Beth Israel Hospital, Boston. The RET proto-oncogene in multiple endocrine neoplasia type 2 and Hirschsprung's disease. N. Engl. J. Med. **335:** 943–951.
28. BORST, M.J., J.M. VANCAMP, M.L. PEACOCK, et al. 1995. Mutational analysis of multiple endocrine neoplasia type 2A associated with Hirschsprung's disease. Surgery **117:** 386–391.
29. DECKER, R.A., & M.L. PEACOCK, 1998. Occurrence of MEN2a in familial Hirschsprung's disease: a new indication for genetic testing of the RET protooncogene. J. Pediatr. Surg. **33:** 207–214.

30. CARNEY, J.A., V.L. GO, G.W. SIZEMORE, et al. 1976. Alimentary-tract ganglioneuromatosis: a major component of the syndrome of multiple endocrine neoplasia type 2b. N. Engl. J. Med. **295:** 1287–1291.
31. MULLIGAN, L.M., C. ENG, C.S. HEALEY, et al. 1994. Specific mutations of the *RET* proto-oncogene are related to disease phenotype in MEN 2A and FMTC. Nat. Genet. **6:** 70–74.
32. TAKAHASHI, M., J. RITZ & G.M. COOPER. 1985. Activation of a novel human transforming gene, ret, by DNA rearrangement. Cell **42:** 581–588.
33. TAKAHASHI, M. 2001. The GDNF/RET signaling pathway and human diseases. Cytokine Growth Factor Rev. **12:** 361–373.
34. JING, S., D. WEN, Y. YU, et al. 1996. GDNF-induced activation of the RET protein tyrosine kinase is mediated by GDNFR-α, a novel receptor for GDNF. Cell **85:** 1113–1124.
35. TRUPP, M., E. ARENAS, M. FAINZILBER, et al. 1996. Functional receptor for GDNF encoded by the c-ret proto-oncogene. Nature **381:** 785–789.
36. SANTORO, M., F. CARLOMAGNO, A. ROMANO, et al. 1995. Activation of *RET* as a dominant transforming gene by germline mutations of MEN2A and MEN2B. Science **267:** 381–383.
37. SCHUCHARDT, A., V. D'AGATI, L. LARSSON-BLOMBERG, et al. 1994. Defects in the kidney and enteric nervous system of mice lacking the tyrosine kinase receptor ret. Nature **367:** 380–382.
38. MANIE, S., M. SANTORO, A. FUSCO, et al. 2001. The RET receptor: function in development and dysfunction in congenital malformation. Trends Genet. **17:** 580–589.
39. DELELLIS, R., H.J. WOLFE, R.F. GAGEL, et al. 1976. Adrenal medullary hyperplasia. Am. J. Pathol. **83:** 177–196.
40. CARNEY, J.A., G.W. SIZEMORE & G.M. TYCE. 1975. Bilateral adrenal medullary hyperplasia in multiple endocrine neoplasia type 2: the precursor of bilateral pheochromocytoma. Mayo Clin. Proc. **50:** 3–10.
41. ZHUANG, Z., W.S. PARK, S. PACK, et al. 1998. Trisomy 7-harboring non-random duplication of the mutant *MET* allele in hereditary papillary renal carcinomas. Nat. Genet. **20:** 66–69.
42. HUANG, S.C., C.A. KOCH, A.O. VORTMEYER, et al. 2000. Duplication of the mutant *RET* allele in trisomy 10 or loss of the wild-type allele in multiple endocrine neoplasia type 2-associated pheochromocytoma. Cancer Res. **60:** 6223–6226.
43. KOCH, C.A., S.C. HUANG, J.F. MOLEY, et al. 2001. Allelic imbalance between the mutant and wild-type *RET* allele in MEN 2A-associated medullary thyroid carcinoma. Oncogene **20:** 7809–7811.
44. COOLEY, L.D., F.F.B. ELDER, A. KNUTH, et al. 1995. Cytogenetic characterization of three human and three rat medullary thyroid carcinoma cell lines. Cancer Genet. Cytogenet. **80:** 138–149.
45. HUANG, S.C. et al. Unpublished data.
46. ZHANG, Z., Y. WANG, H.G. VIKIS, et al. 2001. Wildtype *kras2* can inhibit lung carcinogenesis in mice. Nat. Genet. **29:** 25–33.
47. PFEIFER, G. 2001. A new verdict for an old convict. Nat. Genet **29:** 3–4.
48. KOCH, C.A., S.C. HUANG, A.O. VORTMEYER, et al. 2000. A patient with MEN 2 and multiple mutations of *RET* in the germline. Exp. Clin. Endocrinol. Diabetes **108:** 493.

49. BARTSCH, D.C., C. HASSE, C. SCHUG, et al. 2000. A RET double mutation in the germline of a kindred with FMTC. Exp. Clin. Endocrinol. Diabetes 108: 128–132.
50. TESSITORE, A., A.A. SINISI, D. PASQUALI, et al. 1999. A novel case of multiple endocrine neoplasia type 2A associated with two de novo mutations of the RET protooncogene. J. Clin. Endocrinol. Metab. **84:** 3522–3527.
51. MENKO, F.H., R.B. VAN DER LUIJT, I.A.J. DE VALK, et al. 2002. Atypical MEN 2B associated with two germline RET mutations on the same allele not involving codon 918. J. Clin. Endocrinol. Metab. **87:** 393–397.
52. MULLIGAN, L.M., E. GARDNER, B.A. SMITH, et al. 1993. Genetic events in tumour initiation and progression in multiple endocrine neoplasia type 2. Genes Chromosomes Cancer **6:** 166–177.
53. MOLEY, J.F., M.B. BROTHER, C.T. FONG, et al. 1992. Consistent association of 1p loss of heterozygosity with pheochromocytomas from patients with multiple endocrine neoplasia type 2 syndromes. Cancer Res. **52:** 770.
54. BENN, D.E., T. DWIGHT, A.L. RICHARDSON, et al. 2000. Sporadic and familial pheochromocytomas are associated with loss of at least two discrete intervals on chromosome 1p. Cancer Res. **60:** 7048–7051.
55. DANNENBERG, H., E.J. SPEEL, J. ZHAO, et al. 2000. Losses of chromosomes 1p and 3q are early genetic events in the development of sporadic pheochromocytomas. Am. J. Pathol. **157:** 353–359.
56. KHOSLA, S., V.M. PATEL, I.D. HAY, et al. 1991. Loss of heterozygosity suggests multiple genetic alterations in pheochromocytomas and medullary thyroid carcinomas. J. Clin. Invest. **87:** 1691–1699.
57. ZHUANG, Z., P. BERTHEAU, M.R. EMMERT-BUCK, et al. 1995. A microdissection technique for archival DNA analysis of specific cell populations in less than 1 mm in size. Am. J. Pathol. **146:** 620–625.
58. ZHUANG, Z. & A.O. VORTMEYER. 1998. Applications of tissue microdissection in cancer genetics. Cell Vis. **5:** 43–48
59. THIBODEAU, S.N., N.M. LINDOR, R. HONCHEL, et al. 1994. Mutations in the RET proto-oncogene in sporadic pheochromocytomas. Am. J. Hum. Genet. **55:** A71.
60. HOFSTRA, R.M.W., T. STELWAGEN, R.P. STULP, et al. 1996. Extensive mutation scanning of RET in sporadic medullary thyroid carcinoma and of RET and VHL in sporadic pheochromocytoma reveals involvement of these genes in only a minority of cases. J. Clin. Endocrinol. Metab. **81:** 2881–2884.
61. BAR, M., E. FRIEDMAN, O. JAKOBOVITZ, et al. 1997. Sporadic pheochromocytomas are rarely associated with germline mutations in the von Hippel-Lindau and *RET* genes. Clin. Endocrinol. **47:** 707–712.
62. BRAUCH, H., W. HOPPNER, H. JAHNIG, et al. 1997. Sporadic pheochromocytomas are rarely associated with germline mutations in the *VHL* tumor suppressor gene or the *RET* protooncogene. J. Clin. Endocrinol. Metab. **82:** 4101–4104.
63. LINDOR, N.M., R. HONCHEL, S. KHOSLA, et al. 1995. Mutations in the RET proto-oncogene in sporadic pheochromocytomas. J. Clin. Endocrinol. Metab. **80:** 627–629.
64. BELDJORD, C., F. DESCLAUX-ARRAMOND, M. RAFFIN-SANSON, et al. 1995. The RET protooncogene in sporadic pheochromocytomas: frequent MEN 2-like mutations and new molecular defects. J. Clin. Endocrinol. Metab. 80: 2063–2067.

65. JANUSZEWICZ, A., H.P. NEUMANN, J. LON, *et al.* 2000. Incidence and clinical relevance of *RET* protooncogene germline mutations in pheochromocytoma patients. J. Hypertens. **18:** 1019–1023.
66. KOMMINOTH, P., J. ROTH, S. MULETTA, *et al.* 1996. RET proto-oncogene point mutations in sporadic neuroendocrine tumors. J. Clin. Endocrinol. Metab. **81:** 2–41-6
67. CHEW, S.L., P. LAVENDER, A. JAIN, *et al.* 1995. Absence of mutations in the MEN 2A region of the ret protooncogene in non MEN 2A pheochromocytomas. Clin. Endocrinol. **42:** 17–21.
68. CROSSEY, P.A., C. ENG, M. GINALSKA-MALINOWSKA, *et al.* 1995. Molecular genetic diagnosis of von Hippel-Lindau disease. J. Med. Genet. **32:** 885–886.
69. KOCH, C.A., S.C. HUANG, Z. ZHUANG, *et al.* 2002. Somatic *VHL* gene deletion and point mutation in MEN 2A-associated pheochromocytoma. Oncogene **21:** 479–482
70. KONDO, K. & W.G. KAELIN. 2001. The von Hippel-Lindau tumor suppressor gene. Exp. Cell Res. **264:** 117–125.
71. NEUMANN, H.P. & O.D. WIESTLER. 1991. Clustering of features of von Hippel-Lindau syndrome: evidence for a complex genetic locus. Lancet **337:** 1052–1054.
72. MAHER, E.R., J.R. YATES, R. HARRIES, *et al.* 1990. Clinical features and natural history of von Hippel-Lindau disease. Quart. J. Med. **77:** 1151–1163.
73. RICHARD, S., D. CHAVEAU, Y. CHRETIEN, *et al.* 1994. Renal lesions and pheochromocytoma in von Hippel-Lindau disease. Adv. Nephrol. **23:** 1–27.
74. NEUMANN, H.P., D.P. BERGER, G. SIGMUND, *et al.* 1993. Pheochromocytomas, multiple endocrine neoplasia type 2, and von Hippel-Lindau disease. N. Engl. J. Med. **329:** 1531–1538.
75. CROSSEY, P.A., F.M. RICHARDS, K. FOSTER, *et al.* 1994. Identification of intragenic mutations in the von Hippel-Lindau disease tumor suppressor gene and correlations with disease phenotype. Human Mol. Genet. **3:** 1303–1308.
76. RITTER, M.M., A. FRILLING, P.A. CROSSEY, *et al.* 1996. Isolated familial pheochromocytoma as a variant of von Hippel-Lindau disease. J. Clin. Endocrinol. Metab. **81:** 1035–1037.
77. ZBAR, B., T. KISHIDA, F. CHEN, *et al.* 1996. Germline mutations in the Von Hippel-Lindau disease (VHL) gene in families from North America, Europe, and Japan. Hum. Mutat. **8:** 348–357.
78. BRAUCH, H., T. KISHIDA, D. GLAVAC, *et al.* 1995. Von Hippel-Lindau disease with pheochromocytoma in the Black Forest region of Germany: evidence for a founder effect. Hum. Genet. **95:** 551–556.
79. GROSS, D.J., N. AVISHAI, V. MEINER, *et al.* 1996. Familial pheochromocytoma associated with a novel mutation in the von Hippel-Lindau gene. J. Clin. Endocrinol. Metab. **81:** 147–149.
80. DUAN, D.R., A. PAUSE, W.H. BURGESS, *et al.* 1995. Inhibition of transcription elongation by the VHL tumor suppressor protein. Science **269:** 1402–1407.
81. ASO, T., W.S. LANE, J.W. CONAWAY, *et al.* 1995. Elongin: a multisubunit regulator of elongation by RNA polymerase II. Science **269:** 1439–1443.
82. VORTMEYER, A.O., S.C. HUANG, S.D. PACK, *et al.* 2002. Somatic point mutation of the wildtype allele detected in tumors of patients with *VHL* germline deletion. Oncogene **21:** 1167–1170.
83. NEUMANN, H.P.H., S. GLASKER, B.U. BENDER, *et al.* 2001. Molecular classification of 270 patients with symptomatic pheochromocytoma. [abstract].

84. CHEN, F., T. KISHIDA & M. YAO. 1995. Germline mutations in the von Hippel-Lindau disease tumor suppressor gene: correlations with phenotype. Hum. Mutat. **5:** 66–75.
85. ZEIGER, M.A., B. ZBAR, H. KEISER, et al. 1995. Loss of heterozygosity on the short arm of chromosome 3 in sporadic, von Hippel-Lindau disease-associated, and familial pheochromocytoma. Genes Chromosomes Cancer 13: 151–156.
86. LUBENSKY, I.A., J.R. GNARRA, P. BERTHEAU, et al. 1996. Allelic deletion of the VHL gene detected in multiple microscopic clear cell renal lesions in von Hippel-Lindau disease patients. Am. J. Pathol. **149:** 2089–2094
87. GUTMANN, D.H. & F.S. COLLINS. 1998. Neurofibromatosis type 1. In The Genetic Basis of Human Cancer. B. Vogelstein & K.W. Kinzler, Eds. :443–442. McGraw-Hill. New York.
88. RICCARDI, V.M. 1991. Von Recklinghausen neurofibromatosis. N. Engl. J. Med. **305:** 1617–1627.
89. STACEY, D. & A. KAZLAUSKAS. 2002 Regulation of *RAS* signaling by the cell cycle. Curr. Opin. Genet. Dev. **12:** 44–46.
90. JACKS, T., T.S. SHIH, E.M. SCHMITT, et al. 1994. Tumour predisposition in mice heterozygous for a targeted mutation in NF1. Nat. Genet. **7:** 353–361.
91. XU, W., L.M. MULLIGAN, M.A. PONDER, et al. 1992. Loss of NF1 alleles in pheochromocytomas from patients with type1 neurofibromatosis. Genes Chrom. Cancer **4:** 337–342.
92. GUTMANN D.H., J.L. COLE, W.J. STONE, et al. 1994. Loss of neurofibromin in adrenal gland tumors from patients with neurofibromatosis type 1. Genes Chromosomes Cancer **10:** 55–58.
93. GUTMANN, D.H., R.T. GEIST, K. ROSE, et al. 1995 Loss of neurofibromatosis type 1 gene expression in pheochromocytomas from patients without NF1. Genes Chromosomes Cancer **13:** 104–109.
94. OOSTERWIJK, J.C., J.C. JANSEN, E.M. VAN SCHOTHORST, et al. 1996. First experiences with genetic counselling based on predictive DNA diagnosis in hererditary glomus tumors (paragangliomas). J. Med. Genet. **33:** 379–383.
95. ERICKSON, D., Y.C. KUDVA, M.J. EBERSOLD, et al. 2001. Benign paragangliomas: clinical presentation and treatment outcomes in 236 patients. J. Clin. Endocrinol. Metab. **86:** 5210–5216.
96. KOCH, C.A., K. PACAK & G.P. CHROUSOS. 2002. Endocrine tumors. In Principles and Practice of Pediatric Oncology, 4th ed. P.A. Pizzo & D.G. Poplack, Eds. :1115–1146. Lippincott Williams & Wilkins. Philadelphia, PA.
97. KOCH, C.A., N. AZUMI, M.A. FURLONG, et al. 1999. Carcinoid syndrome caused by an atypical carcinoid of the uterine cervix. J. Clin. Endocrinol. Metab. **84:** 4209–4213.
98. ARIAS-STELLA, J. & J. VALCARCEL. 1973. The human carotid body at high altitudes. Pathol. Microbiol. **39:** 292–297.
99. PACHECO-OJEDA, L., E. DURANGO, C. RODRIQUEZ, et al. 1988. Carotid body tumors at high altitudes: Quito, Ecuador, 1987. World J. Surg. **12:** 856–860.
100. EDWARDS, C., D. HEATH & P. HARRIS. 1971. The carotid body in emphysema and left ventricular hypertrophy. J. Pathol. **104:** 1–13.
101. LACK, E.E. 1978. Hyperplasia of vagal and carotid body paraganglia in patients with chronic hypoxemia. Am. J. Pathol. **91:** 497–516.

102. LACK, E.E. 1977. Carotid body hypertrophy in patients with cystic fibrosis and cyanotic congenital heart disease. Hum. Pathol. **8:** 39–51.
103. BOERSMA, H.H., J.W. WENSING, T.L. KHO, *et al.* 2002 Compensatory uptake of I-123 MIBG in the contralateral adrenal gland after removal of a pheochromocytoma. Clin. Nucl. Med. **27:** 113–116.
104. BAYSAL, B.E., J.E. WILLET-BROZICK, P.E. TASCHNER, *et al.* 2001. A high-resolution integrated map spanning the SDHD gene at 11q23: a 1.1-Mb BAC contig, a partial transcript map and fifteen new repeat polymorphisms in a tumor suppressor region. Eur. J. Hum. Genet. **9:** 121–129.
105. MARIMAN, E.C., S.E. VAN BEERSUM, C.W. CREMERS, *et al.* 1995. Fine mapping of a putatively imprinted gene for familial nonchromaffin paragangliomas to chromosome 11q13.1: evidence for genetic heterogeneity. Hum. Genet. **95:** 56–62.
106. DEVILEE, P., E.M. VAN SCHOTHORST, A.F. BARDOEL, *et al.* 1994. Allelotype of head and neck paragangliomas: allelic imbalance is confined to the long arm of chromosome 11, the site of the predisposing locus PGL. Genes Chromosomes Cancer **11:** 71–78.
107. VAN SCHOTHORST, E.M., M. BEEKMAN, P. TORREMANS, *et al.* 1998. Paragangliomas of the head and neck region show complete loss of heterozygosity at 11q22–23 in chief cells and the flow-sorted DNA aneuploid fraction. Hum. Pathol. **29:** 1045–1049.
108. VARGAS, M.P., Z. ZHUANG, C. WANG, *et al.* 1997. Loss of heterozygosity on the short arm of chromosomes 1 and 3 in sporadic pheochromocytoma and extraadrenal paraganglioma. Hum. Pathol. **28:** 411–415.
109. TSUTSUMI, M., Y. YOKOTA, T. KAKIZOE, *et al.* 1989. Loss of heterozygosity on chromosome 1p and 11p in sporadic pheochromocytoma. J. Natl. Cancer Inst. **81:** 367–370.
110. MATHEW, C.G.P., K.S. CHIN, D.F. EASTON, *et al.* 1987. A linked genetic marker for multiple endocrine neoplasia type 2A on chromosome 10. Nature **328:** 528–530.
111. RODIEN, P., X. JEUNEMAITRE, C. DUMONT, *et al.* 1997. Genetic alterations of the RET proto-oncogene in familial and sporadic pheochromocytomas. Horm. Res. **47:** 263–268.
112. NEUMANN, H.P. *et al.* 2002. Germline mutations in nonsyndromic pheochromocytoma. N. Engl. J. Med. **346:** 1486–1488.

New Advances in the Biochemical Diagnosis of Pheochromocytoma

Moving beyond Catecholamines

JACQUES W.M. LENDERS,[a] KAREL PACAK,[b] AND GRAEME EISENHOFER[c]

[a]*Department of Internal Medicine, St. Radboud University Medical Center, Nijmegen, the Netherlands*

[b]*Pediatric and Reproductive Endocrinology Branch, National Institute of Child Health and Human Development, National Institutes of Health, Bethesda, Maryland 20892, USA*

[c]*Clinical Neurocardiology Section, National Institute of Neurological Disorders and Stroke, National Institutes of Health, Bethesda, Maryland 20892, USA*

ABSTRACT: Pheochromocytomas are dangerous tumors that, although a rare cause of hypertension, require consideration among large numbers of patients. The resulting low prevalence of the tumor among tested populations and the inadequacies of commonly used biochemical tests make excluding or confirming the tumor an often difficult and time-consuming task. Recognition that catecholamines are metabolized to free metanephrines within pheochromocytoma tumor cells, and that this process is independent of catecholamine release, provides a rationale for use of these metabolites in the biochemical diagnosis of pheochromocytoma. Here we briefly review the history of biochemical diagnosis of pheochromocytoma in relation to recent data about the diagnostic utility of plasma free metanephrines for detection of these tumors. Measurements of urinary or plasma catecholamines have reasonable sensitivity for detection of most pheochromocytomas, particularly those in patients with sustained hypertension. False-negative test results can, however, occur in asymptomatic patients tested because of an adrenal incidentaloma or a familial predisposition for pheochromocytoma, or when sampling is carried out between episodes of paroxysmal hypertension. Measurements of urinary total metanephrines or vanillylmandelic acid are less reliable and are of little value as initial screening tests. In contrast, measurements of plasma concentrations or free metanephrines or 24-hour urinary outputs of fractionated normetanephrine and metanephrine almost always reveal the tumor.

Address for correspondence: Graeme Eisenhofer, Building 10, Room 6N252, National Institutes of Health, 10 Center Drive, MSC-1620, Bethesda, MD 20892-1620. Voice: 301-496-8925; fax: 301-402-0180.
ge@box-g.nih.gov

Ann. N.Y. Acad. Sci. 970: 29–40 (2002). © 2002 New York Academy of Sciences.

Although, both tests have similarly high sensitivity, the relatively low specificity of urinary fractionated metanephrines means that pheochromocytomas can be more efficiently excluded or confirmed using measurements of plasma free metanephrines.

KEYWORDS: pheochromocytoma; normetanephrine; metanephrine; norepinephrine; epinephrine; diagnosis, adrenal incidentaloma, von Hippel–Lindau disease; multiple endocrine neoplasia type 2

THE HISTORICAL PERSPECTIVE

Recognition that the clinical features of pheochromocytoma are largely due to excess catecholamine secretion provided the basis for early biochemical tests involving bioassays and then fluorometric assays of catecholamines in alumina extracts of urine.[1,2] Subsequent findings of high levels of certain catecholamine metabolites in the urine of patients with pheochromocytoma led to colorimetric assays of vanillylmandelic acid (VMA) and metanephrines as additional diagnostic markers of the tumor.[3,4] The metanephrines, normetanephrine and metanephrine, are the O-methylated metabolites of norepinephrine and epinephrine, whereas VMA represents the final end-product of norepinephrine and epinephrine metabolism. The much higher urinary concentrations of these metabolites than of the parent amines provides an advantage to measurements of metanephrines and VMA compared to catecholamines. Perhaps due to this, the largely outmoded colorimetric assays of urinary VMA and total metanephrines persist as routine methods for tumor diagnosis.

The above assays of total metanephrines, VMA, and catecholamines performed on samples of urine and tumor tissue led Crout and Sjoerdsma to conclude that catecholamines were metabolized substantially within tumors before reaching the circulation.[5] The importance of these observations, however, remained largely ignored, perhaps in part due to the emergence of radioenzymatic and high-pressure liquid chromatography (HPLC) assays sensitive enough for reliable detection of catecholamines in plasma and urine. Since pheochromocytomas are characterized by excess catecholamine production, and since it is the secretion of catecholamines that causes the hypertension and symptoms characteristic of these tumors, measuring plasma or urinary catecholamines for diagnosis of pheochromocytoma seems entirely logical. Indeed, over the ensuing decades application of catecholamine assays have become the mainstay for biochemical detection of pheochromocytoma, with several reports attesting to the good overall diagnostic utility of these measurements.[6–8]

The development of radiological methods for tumor localization in the 1980s considerably improved diagnosis of pheochromocytoma and also led to recognition of adrenal incidentalomas as a new clinical problem.[9] Increasing recognition of hereditary factors as causes of some forms of pheochromocytoma and advancements in molecular genetics for diagnosis of these familial syndromes led to recommendations that such patients be screened for pheochromocytoma on a periodic basis.[10,11] The foregoing developments have increasingly led to detection of pheochromocytomas where the tumor would not have otherwise been considered. Thus, pheochromocytomas associated with adrenal incidentalomas or hereditary cancer syndromes, such as multiple endocrine neoplasia type 2 (MEN-2) or von Hippel–Lindau (VHL) disease, are now being routinely found in patients who are completely asymptomatic and normotensive.[9,11–15] In these patients the tumors are often small and do not secrete large amounts of catecholamines, presenting a challenge for biochemical diagnosis.

The advances in genetic and radiological techniques that are allowing improved recognition of at-risk patients are therefore now severely testing the diagnostic limits of available biochemical tests for pheochromocytoma. In particular, urinary or plasma levels of catecholamines can often be normal in patients with pheochromocytoma who are asymptomatic and normotensive, or when sampling is carried out between episodes in patients who have paroxysmal hypertension.[14–16] It has also become increasingly clear that measurements of VMA in 24-hour urine samples do not provide a sensitive method for detection of pheochromocytoma.[14,17–19]

ADVANCES IN DIAGNOSIS: FOCUS ON THE METANEPHRINES

Today's tests of catecholamine excess used to diagnose pheochromocytoma include measurements of catecholamines and metanephrines in urine or plasma and VMA in urine (TABLE 1). Colorimetric measurements of total metanephrines, representing the sum of normetanephrine and metanephrine determined together as a single analyte, have been superseded by HPLC measurements of fractionated normetanephrine and metanephrine.[20] Liquid chromatography coupled with mass spectrometry represents a more recent advance that offers higher analytical specificity, thereby avoiding many of the pitfalls associated with drug or dietary interferences.[21] For measurements of urinary metanephrines, whether they be determined as total or fractionated metanephrines, there is usually a deconjugation step. This step liberates free metanephrines from the much higher concentrations of sulfate-conjugated metanephrines. Importantly, the sulfate-conjugated metanephrines are different metabolites from the free metanephrines and are produced in different parts of the body, particularly the gastrointestinal tract.[22,23]

Measurements of metanephrines in plasma represent another advance. At first these assays were mainly carried out after a deconjugation step.[24,25]

TABLE 1. Biochemical tests of catecholamine excess for diagnosis of pheochromocytoma

Biochemical test (assay method)	Upper reference limits[a] (true negatives ≫ false negatives)	Tumor possible (false positives > true positives)	Tumor likely (true positives ≫ false positives)
Urine tests			
1. Catecholamines (HPLC)			
Norepinephrine (μg/24 hr)	80	>80 and <300	>300
Epinephrine (μg/24 h)	20	>20 and <50	>50
2. Fractionated metanephrines (HPLC)[b]			
Normetanephrine (μg/24 hr)	540/310	>540 and <1400	>1400
Metanephrine (μg/24 hr)	240/140	>240 and <1000	>1000
3. Total metanephrines (spectrophotometry)			
Sum of NMN and MN (mg/24 hr)	1.2	>1.2 and <2	>2
4. Vanillymandelic acid (spectrophotometry)			
VMA (mg/24 hr)	7.9	>7.9 and <12	>12
Blood tests			
5. Catecholamines (HPLC)			
Norepinephrine (pg/mL)	498	>498 and <2000	>2000
Epinephrine (pg/mL)	83	>83 and <400	>400
6. Free metanephrines (HPLC)			
Normetanephrine (pg/mL)	112	>112 and <400	>400
Metanephrine (pg/mL)	61	>61 and <220	>220

[a]Upper reference limits vary among different laboratories. Those shown are those in use at the National Institutes of Health, Bethesda, Maryland, USA.

[b]Upper reference limits for urinary fractionated metanephrines are shown separately for men and women.

Thus, similar to the assays in urine, such measurements in plasma mainly reflect concentrations of normetanephrine-sulfate and metanephrine-sulfate. These sulfate-conjugates are present in plasma in 20- to 30-fold–high concentrations than levels of the free metabolites.[26] This makes the deconjugated metabolites much easier to measure than the free metanephrines and represents the single major advantage of the former over the latter measurements.

It is, however, the free metanephrines that are produced in large amounts within adrenal medullary chromaffin or pheochromocytoma tumor cells.[26–28] This production occurs secondary to catecholamines leaking from storage granules into the cytoplasm where the presence of the enzyme, catechol-*O*-methyltransferase, leads to conversion of norepinephrine to normetanephrine and of epinephrine to metanephrine. More than 90% of circulating metanephrine and between 24% and 40% of circulating normetanephrine are thereby produced within the adrenal glands.[26,27] In patients with pheochromocytoma more than 90% of the elevated plasma concentrations of free metanephrines are produced within tumor tissue, and this production is continuous and independent of catecholamine release.[28] These considerations provide the theoretical basis of why measurements of plasma free metanephrines provide advantages over measurements of catecholamines and other metabolites for diagnosis of pheochromocytoma.[23]

The radioenzymatic assay of plasma free normetanephrine developed by DeQuattro and colleagues was perhaps the first to provide data hinting at the possible utility of these measurements for diagnosis of pheochromocytoma.[29] These investigators also established that substantial amounts of normetanephrine were produced within tumors and secreted into the bloodstream. Later development of an HPLC method for measurement of both normetanephrine and metanephrine[30] subsequently led to findings that first established the high sensitivity of plasma free metanephrines for detection of pheochromocytoma.[31] This initial study was followed by several more that confirmed the high sensitivity of plasma free metanephrines for detection of pheochromocytomas found during routine screening of patients with MEN-2 and VHL disease,[14] or discovered as an incidentaloma[15] or because of suspicious signs and symptoms.[32]

Up until the turn of the 21st century, all studies examining biochemical tests used for diagnosis of pheochromocytoma suffered from at least one and, in most cases, several limitations. These included small numbers of patients, limited comparisons of available biochemical tests, and inappropriate comparison groups for establishing specificity.[6,8,14,17–19,31–37] Where studies did include appropriate comparison groups of patients without pheochromocytoma, the criteria for exclusion of the tumor was often unclear. Thus, the test or combination of tests that provides the best method for diagnosis of pheochromocytoma remained largely unsettled.

WHICH TEST IS BEST?

To definitively establish the best test for biochemical diagnosis of pheochromocytoma we carried out a multi-center, largely prospective study involving large numbers of patients tested because of suggestive signs and

TABLE 2. Sensitivities and specificities of biochemical tests for diagnosis of pheochromocytoma

	Sensitivity	Specificity
Plasma free metanephrines	99% (211/214)	89% (575/644)
Plasma catecholamines	84% (178/212)	81% (523/643)
Urine fractionated metanephrines	97% (102/105)	69 % (310/452)
Urine catecholamines	86% (151/175)	88% (471/535)
Urine total metanephrines	77% (88/114)	93% (170/183)
Urine vanillylmandelic acid	64% (96/151)	95% (442/465)

NOTE: The reference limits used to calculate sensitivity and specificity are presented in TABLE 1.
The sensitivities of tests of plasma free and urinary fractionated metanephrines or plasma and urinary catecholamines were determined as the percentage of patients with pheochromocytoma with positive test results for either normetanephrine or metanephrine (i.e., for tests of plasma or urinary metanephrines) or with positive test results for either norepinephrine or epinephrine (i.e., for tests of plasma or urinary catecholamines).

symptoms, a finding of an adrenal incidentaloma, or a predisposition to develop the tumor because of hereditary factors or a previous history of the tumor. Biochemical tests included measurements of plasma and urinary catecholamines, urinary fractionated metanephrines, urinary total metanephrines, urinary VMA, and plasma concentrations of free metanephrines. Selection of patients in the final analyses was based on whether pheochromocytoma could be excluded or confirmed by standard criteria that were necessarily independent of the diagnostic biochemical tests being evaluated. Pheochromocytoma was thereby confirmed in 214 patients and excluded in 644 patients. The methodological details and results of the study are reported in detail elsewhere,[38] but are also summarized here (TABLE 2).

Our findings confirmed those of other reports that measurements of plasma free metanephrines or urinary fractionated metanephrines offer higher sensitivity for diagnosis of pheochromocytoma than measurements of plasma or urinary catecholamines or of urinary total metanephrines or VMA.[14,18,31,32,37] The high sensitivity of plasma free metanephrines and urinary fractionated metanephrines means that a negative result for either test excludes the presence of all but the smallest of pheochromocytomas.

Only three of 214 patients had normal levels of plasma free metanephrines despite a tumor. These false-negative results were observed in two asymptomatic and normotensive patients with hereditary pheochromocytoma and one patient with metastatic pheochromocytoma diagnosed 3½ years after the tests of metanephrines were run and 13 years after removal of the primary tumor. In such patients testing should be carried out at periodic intervals regardless of suspicious signs and symptoms. In other patients with hypertension and symptoms—and where there is no risk from hereditary factors or previous history—a negative result for tests of plasma free or urinary fractionated metanephrines excludes pheochromocytoma so that no further testing should be necessary. Of importance, this conclusion is based on the upper reference limits used in our study (TABLE 1). Use of higher upper reference limits may lead to higher specificity, but with a loss of sensitivity and an increased possibility of a missed diagnosis.

Although tests of plasma free metanephrines and urinary fractionated metanephrines had similarly high sensitivity, the specificity of the latter test was relatively poor (TABLE 2). This means that a positive result for plasma free metanephrines is more predictive of a pheochromocytoma than a positive result for urinary fractionated metanephrines. More importantly, this also means that tests of plasma free metanephrines exclude pheochromocytoma in many more patients without the tumor than do tests of urinary fractionated metanephrines. Thus, among all five tests that were examined, including urinary fractionated metanephrines, measurements of plasma free metanephrines provide the best test for excluding or confirming pheochromocytoma.

What difference does a positive or negative result mean in terms of probabilities of having or not having a pheochromocytoma? As shown in FIGURE 1 this depends importantly on the pretest probability or prevalence of the tumor among the tested population, which can vary considerably depending on clinical presentation. In patients tested because of hypertension the pre-test probability of the tumor is less than 1%, whereas in patients who also have a familial history or the finding of an adrenal mass, the pre-test probability is higher. For all biochemical tests the larger increases in probability of having a pheochromocytoma after a positive result occur at lower pre-test probabilities (FIG. 1). These effects taper off at high pre-test probabilities where differences between tests dissipate. For negative results for plasma free metanephrines or urinary fractionated metanephrines, the percentage increases in post-test probabilities of not having a pheochromocytoma continuously get larger at higher pre-test probabilities, whereas those for other tests do not.

Apart from variations in pre-test prevalence, use of positive and negative predictive values for determining the probability or likelihood of a pheochromocytoma do not take into account the absolute value of a test result and may vary depending on the reference limits in use by different laboratories. These are limitations that can be particularly misleading when comparing the performance of various diagnostic tests. For example, the higher specificities and positive predictive values of tests of urinary total metanephrine and VMA might suggest that elevated values for these tests provide a better way to confirm a pheochromocytoma than elevated levels of plasma free metanephrines. This conclusion, however, is incorrect. By increasing the upper reference limits for normetanephrine from 112 pg/mL to 400 pg/mL and for metanephrine from 61 pg/mL to 220 pg/mL the specificity of the test of plasma free metanephrines increases from 89% to 100% and the sensitivity decreases from 99% to 79%. Even at these higher upper reference limits the sensitivity for plasma free metanephrines remains higher than that for urinary VMA (79%

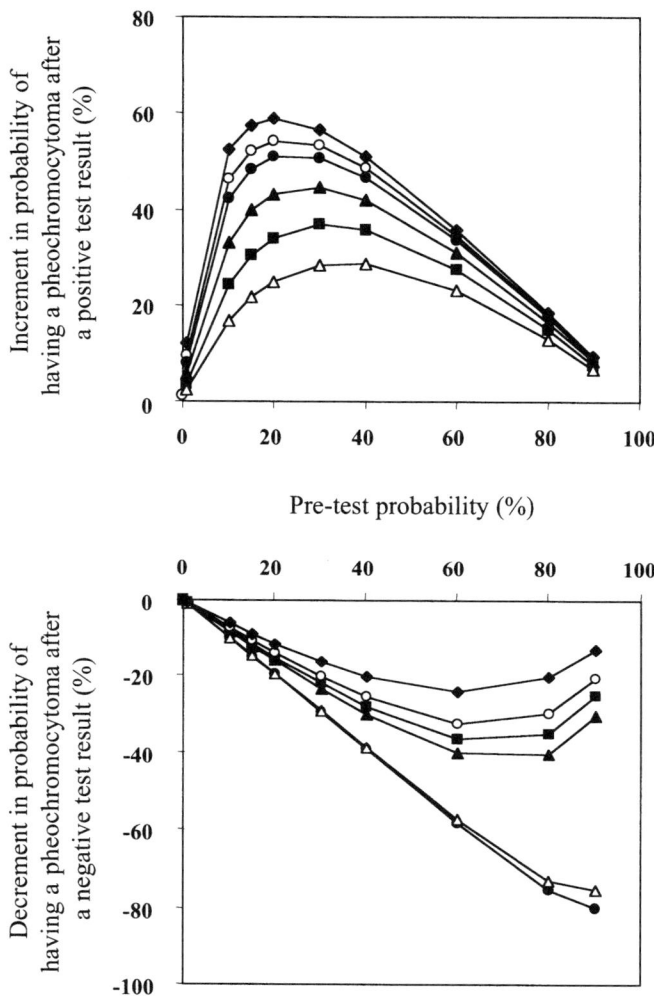

FIGURE 1. Relationships between pre-test probability (prevalence) of a pheochromocytoma and the change in probability of the tumor after biochemical testing. The *upper panel* shows the effects of a positive test result on the probability of having a pheochromocytoma as a function of pretest probability of pheochromocytoma (i.e., prevalence). The *lower panel* shows the effects of a negative test result on the probability of not having a pheochromocytoma as a function of pre-test probability of pheochromocytoma (i.e., prevalence). Results are shown for plasma free metanephrines (●), plasma catecholamines (■), urinary fractionated metanephrines (△), urinary total metanephrines (○), urinary catecholamines (▲), and urinary VMA (◆).

versus 64%). Also, the specificity and positive predictive value of plasma free metanephrines are not only higher than for urinary VMA, but the test also positively confirms more cases of pheochromocytoma than does use of VMA.

The foregoing considerations illustrate that at least 79% of patients with pheochromocytoma can be expected to have elevations of plasma free normetanephrine exceeding 400 pg/mL or of metanephrine exceeding 220 pg/mL. In these patients the extent of increase in plasma free normetanephrine or metanephrine indicates the presence of a pheochromocytoma with extremely high probability so that other biochemical tests may not be necessary. In such patients, localization of the tumor by imaging studies becomes the priority.

An elevated plasma free normetanephrine between 112 to 400 pg/mL or of metanephrine between 61 to 220 pg/mL remains equivocal. Such patients may or may not have a pheochromocytoma. Because of the low prevalence of pheochromocytoma in a given tested population it is likely that the number of false-positive test results with values within the above ranges will far exceed the number of true-positive test results. These patients therefore remain a challenge to diagnosis and invariably require additional testing.

CONCLUSIONS

Advances in current understanding of catecholamine metabolism provide a theoretical basis for why measurements of plasma free metanephrines offer advantages over other biochemical tests used for diagnosis of pheochromocytoma. Plasma concentrations of free normetanephrine below 112 pg/mL (0.61 nmol/L) and metanephrine below 61 pg/mL (0.31 nmol/L) in a patient tested because of hypertension and suspicious symptoms reliably exclude pheochromocytoma so that no other tests for the tumor should be necessary. However, most patients with pheochromocytoma have increases of plasma normetanephrine above 400 pg/mL (2.2 nmol/L) and/or of metanephrine above 220 pg/ml (1.1 nmol/L). In these patients the magnitudes of increase are sufficient for reliable confirmation of a pheochromocytoma so that the immediate task is to locate the tumor. Since the test of plasma free metanephrines eliminates the need for multiple screening tests and is likely to reduce the unnecessary use of follow-up tests, including expensive imaging studies, use of this test not only improves diagnosis of pheochromocytoma, but achieves this at less cost.

REFERENCES

1. ENGEL, A. & U.S. VON EULER. 1950. Diagnostic value of increased urinary output of noradrenaline and adrenaline in phaeochromocytoma. Lancet **2:** 387.

2. GOLDENBERG, M., I. SERLIN, T. EDWARDS, *et al.* 1954. Chemical screening methods for the diagnosis of pheochromocytoma. Am. J. Med. **16:** 310–328.
3. SJOERDSMA, A., L.C. LEEPER, L.L. TERRY, *et al.* 1959. Studies on the biogenesis and metabolism of norepinephrine in patients with pheochromocytoma. J. Clin. Invest. **38:** 31–38.
4. GITLOW, S.E., M. MENDLOWITZ, S. KHASSIS, *et al.* 1960. The diagnosis of pheochromocytoma by determination of urinary 3-methoxy-4-hydroxymandelic acid. J. Clin. Invest. **39:** 221–226.
5. CROUT, J.R. & A. SJOERDSMA. 1964. Turnover and metabolism of catecholamines in patients with pheochromocytoma. J. Clin. Invest. **43:** 94–102.
6. BRAVO, E.L., R.C. TARAZI, R.W. GIFFORD, *et al.* 1979. Circulating and urinary catecholamines in pheochromocytoma. Diagnostic and pathophysiologic implications. N. Engl. J. Med. **301:** 682–686.
7. MANNELLI, M., M.L. DE FEO, M. MAGGI, *et al.* 1987. Usefulness of basal catecholamine plasma levels and clonidine suppression test in the diagnosis of pheochromocytoma. J. Endocrinol. Invest. **10:** 377–382.
8. DUNCAN, M.W., P. COMPTON, L. LAZARUS, *et al.* 1988. Measurement of norepinephrine and 3,4-dihydroxyphenylglycol in urine and plasma for the diagnosis of pheochromocytoma. N. Engl. J. Med. **319:** 136–142.
9. MANTERO, F., M. TERZOLO, G. ARNALDI, *et al.* 2001. A survey on adrenal incidentaloma in Italy: Study Group on Adrenal Tumors of the Italian Society of Endocrinology. J. Clin. Endocrinol. Metab. **85:** 637–644.
10. CALMETTES, C., B.A. PONDER, J.A. FISCHER, *et al.* 1992. Early diagnosis of the multiple endocrine neoplasia type 2 syndrome: consensus statement. European Community Concerted Action: Medullary Thyroid Carcinoma. Eur. J. Clin. Invest. **22:** 755–760.
11. NEUMANN, H.P., D.P. BERGER, G. SIGMUND, *et al.* 1993. Pheochromocytomas, multiple endocrine neoplasia type 2, and von Hippel-Lindau disease. N. Engl. J. Med. **329:** 1531–1538.
12. APRILL, B.S., A.J. DRAKE, D.H. LASSETER, *et al.* 1994. Silent adrenal nodules in von Hippel-Lindau disease suggest pheochromocytoma. Ann. Intern. Med. **120:** 485–487.
13. WALTHER, M.M., R. REITER, H.R. KEISER, *et al.* 1999. Clinical and genetic characterization of pheochromocytoma in von Hippel-Lindau families: comparison with sporadic pheochromocytoma gives insight into natural history of pheochromocytoma. J. Urol. **162:** 659–664.
14. EISENHOFER, G., J.W. LENDERS, W.M. LINEHAN, *et al.* 1999. Plasma normetanephrine and metanephrine for detecting pheochromocytoma in von Hippel-Lindau disease and multiple endocrine neoplasia type 2. N. Engl. J. Med. **340:** 1872–1879.
15. RABER, W., W. RAFFESBERG, E. KMEN, *et al.* 2000. Pheochromocytoma with normal urinary and plasma catecholamines but elevated plasma free metanephrines in a patient with adrenal incidentaloma. Endocrinologist **10:** 65–68.
16. SHAWAR, L. & F. SVEC. 1996. Pheochromocytoma with elevated metanephrines as the only biochemical finding. J. La. State. Med. Soc. **148:** 535–538.
17. PEASTON, R.T. & L.C. LAI. 1993. Biochemical detection of phaechromocytoma: should we still be measuring urinary HMMA? J. Clin. Pathol. **46:** 734–737.

18. GERLO, E.A. & C. SEVENS. 1994. Urinary and plasma catecholamines and urinary catecholamine metabolites in pheochromocytoma: diagnostic value in 19 cases. Clin. Chem. **40:** 250–256.
19. MANNELLI, M., L. IANNI, A. CILOTTI, *et al.* 1999. Pheochromocytoma in Italy: a multicentric retrospective study. Eur. J. Endocrinol. **141:** 619–624.
20. BERTANI-DZIEDZIC, L.M., A.M. KRSTULOVIC, S.W. DZIEDZIC, *et al.* 1981. Analysis of urinary metanephrines by reversed-phase high-performance liquid chromatography and electrochemical detection. Clin. Chim. Acta **110:** 1–8.
21. TAYLOR, R.L. & R.J. SINGH. 2002. Validation of liquid chromatography-tandem mass spectrometry method for analysis of urinary conjugated metanephrine and normetanephrine for screening of pheochromocytoma. Clin. Chem. **48:** 533–539.
22. EISENHOFER, G. 2001. Free or total metanephrines for diagnosis of pheochromocytoma: what is the difference? Clin. Chem. **47:** 988–999.
23. EISENHOFER, G., T.-T. HUYNH, M. HIROI, *et al.* 2001. Understanding catecholamine metabolism as a guide to the biochemical diagnosis of pheochromocytoma. Rev. Endocr. Metab. Dis. **2:** 297–311.
24. MORNEX, R., L. PEYRIN, R. PAGLIARI, *et al.* 1991. Measurement of plasma methoxyamines for the diagnosis of pheochromocytoma. Horm. Res. **36:** 220–226.
25. MARINI, M., M. FATHI & M. VALLOTTON. 1994. Determination of serum metanephrines in the diagnosis of pheochromocytoma. Ann. Endocrinol. **54:** 337–342.
26. EISENHOFER, G., P. FRIBERG, K. PACAK, *et al.* 1995. Plasma metadrenalines: do they provide useful information about sympatho-adrenal function and catecholamine metabolism? Clin. Sci. (Colch). **88:** 533–542.
27. EISENHOFER, G., B. RUNDQVIST, A. ANEMAN, *et al.* 1995. Regional release and removal of catecholamines and extraneuronal metabolism to metanephrines. J. Clin. Endocrinol. Metab. **80:** 3009–3017.
28. EISENHOFER, G., H. KEISER, P. FRIBERG, *et al.* 1998. Plasma metanephrines are markers of pheochromocytoma produced by catechol-O-methyltransferase within tumors. J. Clin. Endocrinol. Metab. **83:** 2175–2185.
29. DEQUATTRO, V., P. SULLIVAN, A. FOTI, *et al.* 1980. Central and regional normetadrenaline in evaluation of neurogenic aspects of hypertension: aid to diagnosis of phaeochromocytoma. Clin. Sci. **59:** 275s–277s.
30. LENDERS, J.W.M., G. EISENHOFER, I. ARMANDO, *et al.* 1993. Determination of plasma metanephrines by liquid chromatography with electrochemical detection. Clin. Chem. **39:** 97–103.
31. LENDERS, J.W., H.R. KEISER, D.S. GOLDSTEIN, *et al.* 1995. Plasma metanephrines in the diagnosis of pheochromocytoma. Ann. Intern. Med. **123:** 101–109.
32. RABER, W., W. RAFFESBERG, M. BISCHOF, *et al.* 2000. Diagnostic efficacy of unconjugated plasma metanephrines for the detection of pheochromocytoma. Arch. Intern. Med. **160:** 2957–2963.
33. YOUNG, M.J., C. DMUCHOWSKI, J.W. WALLIS, *et al.* 1989. Biochemical tests for pheochromocytoma: strategies in hypertensive patients. J. Gen. Intern. Med. **4:** 273–276.
34. HERON, E., G. CHATELLIER, E. BILLAUD, *et al.* 1996. The urinary metanephrine-to-creatinine ratio for the diagnosis of pheochromocytoma. Ann. Intern. Med. **125:** 300–303.

35. WITTELES, R.M., E.L. KAPLAN & M.F. ROIZEN. 2000. Sensitivity of diagnostic and localization tests for pheochromocytoma in clinical practice. Arch. Intern. Med. **160:** 2521–2524.
36. HERNANDEZ, F.C., M. SANCHEZ, A. ALVAREZ, et al. 2001. A five-year report on experience in the detection of pheochromocytoma. Clin. Biochem. **33:** 649–655.
37. GARDET, V., B. GATTA, G. SIMONNET, et al. 2001. Lessons from an unpleasant surprise: a biochemical strategy for the diagnosis of pheochromocytoma. J. Hypertens. **19:** 1029–1035.
38. LENDERS, J.W., K. PACAK, M. M. WALTHER, et al. 2002. Biochemical diagnosis of pheochromocytoma: which test is best? JAMA **287:** 1427–1434.

New Therapeutic and Surgical Approaches for Sporadic and Hereditary Pheochromocytoma

McCLELLAN M. WALTHER

Urologic Oncology Branch, DCS/NCI, National Institutes of Health, Bethesda, Maryland 20892-1502, USA

ABSTRACT: Pheochromocytoma is a rare, surgically correctable cause of hypertension. Modern medical blockade has significantly improved patient survival and morbidity. The last decade has seen the identification of the genes responsible for several hereditary causes of pheochromocytoma. Evaluation of these patients has demonstrated different catecholamine profiles associated with the different syndromes. Genetic testing and new, more sensitive catecholamine tests are allowing better, earlier diagnosis of affected patients. Some patients with small tumors deemed nonfunctional by traditional methods may be safely observed until function is demonstrated. Laparoscopic surgery has supplanted the use of open surgery in the management of these tumors. Adrenocortical-sparing surgery may be performed using laparoscopy in patients with hereditary forms of pheochromocytoma.

KEYWORDS: pheochromocytoma; diagnosis; surgery; hereditary disorders

INTRODUCTION

Pheochromocytoma is a rare cause of surgically correctable hypertension. The incidence of sporadic pheochromocytoma has been estimated as 1.55–1.9 per million in the general population per year.[1–3] New approaches important in the clinical and surgical management of pheochromocytoma are presented in this section of the book.

Preoperative medical blockade of pheochromocytoma has historically consisted of alpha- and beta-adrenergic blockade. Combined medical blockade refers to the addition of the catecholamine synthesis inhibitor metyrosine to traditional blockade. This addition has been shown to significantly decrease the amount of catecholamines in the tumors, contributing to better blockade.

Address for correspondence: McClellan M. Walther, M.D., Urologic Oncology Branch, DCS/NCI/NIH, Building 10, Room 2B-43, 10 Center Drive, MSC 1502, Bethesda, MD 20892-1502. Voice: 301-402-2251; fax: 301-402-0922.
macw@nih.gov

Alternatively, calcium channel blockers have also been proposed as a quicker, equally efficacious regimen. After adequate pharmacological blockade, the use of laparoscopic surgery has resulted in marked decrease in morbidity with no increased risk compared to open surgery.

A number of hereditary forms of pheochromocytoma and the genes that cause them have been identified or localized by linkage analysis. Screening family members clinically or with genetic testing can identify patients with small tumors that are often nonfunctional by traditional testing. Observation of these small tumors has been performed until they become functional, often avoiding surgery for years in young otherwise healthy patients. When surgery is indicated, laparoscopic partial adrenalectomy has been performed to avoid the morbidity associated with medical adrenal replacement. New data suggest that the addition of dehydroepiandrosterone to standard medical adrenal replacement may improve patients' bone quality and quality of life.

MEDICAL BLOCKADE

Preoperative Blockade

Pheochromocytomas are unpredictable in nature and minimal tumor stimulation can be associated with a massive outpouring of catecholamines, resulting in hypertensive crisis, arrhythmias, or stroke. Induction of anesthesia and surgical resection without catecholamine blockade has been associated with a 24–50% mortality. The development of medical catecholamine blockade and modern anesthesia techniques has resulted in a significant decrease in mortality.

Modern biochemical blockade for pheochromocytoma has primarily consisted of three regimens: alpha- and beta-adrenergic blockade alone, alpha- and beta-adrenergic blockade accompanied with the use of a catecholamine synthesis inhibitor, or calcium channel blockade.

Alpha- and Beta-adrenergic Blockade

Phenoxybenzamine (starting at 10 mg every 12 hours for adults, for 2 weeks prior to surgery) provides long-acting, nonselective, alpha-adrenergic blockade, contributing to vascular dilation with expansion of constricted fluid volume. The dosage can be increased 0.5 mg/kg/day in two divided doses as needed to control blood pressure or symptoms. A final preoperative dose (1 mg/kg) is given at midnight the night before surgery. After this dose is administered, patients are placed at bed rest with the side rails up because of associated orthostatic hypotension. Somnolence, headache, and nasal congestion can be associated with this regimen. A disadvantage of this blockade is that it can take about 2 weeks to reach maximum effect.

Nonspecific blockade affecting alpha-2 receptors can lead to loss of feedback inhibition in cardiac sympathetic nerve endings with resultant tachycardia. A beta-adrenergic blocker is added as needed to control this reflex tachycardia (pulse greater than 100). Beta blockade has also been useful in blunting tachycardia related to epinephrine-secreting tumors. Labetalol, with alpha- and beta-blockade action (gradually titrated to as high as 1600 mg per day), can be useful in beta-blockade. Administration of a beta-blocker before alpha blockade can worsen hypertension secondary to unopposed vasoconstriction. Care must also be taken in patients with a history of obstructive lung disease or peripheral vascular disease. Use of specific alpha-1-adrenergic blockade has recently been used to avoid these side effects.

Combined Medical Blockade

The addition of metyrosine to alpha- and beta-adrenergic blockade is termed combined medical blockade; both catecholamine synthesis and end-organ effectors are blocked. Metyrosine is a competitive inhibitor of the enzyme tyrosine hydroxylase, the rate-limiting enzyme in catecholamine production, blocking the conversion of tyrosine to DOPA.[4] The use of metyrosine over two weeks decreases tumor catecholamine content by 50–80%. In adults, metyrosine is administered as a dose of 250 mg every 6 hours. After one week the dosage is increased by 250 mg to 500 mg every two to three days as needed for additional blockade. A preoperative dose of 1 gram is given at midnight the night before surgery.

The addition of metyrosine to preoperative blockade has resulted in less medication required to control blood pressure, lower intraoperative fluid requirements, and less blood loss.[5] About 10% of patients develop excessive sedation, depression, hallucinations, sleep disturbances, extrapyramidal signs, or tremor. Sinemet has been used with some success to control these symptoms. Doses greater than 4 gm per day have been associated with the development of metyrosine crystaluria. The use of combined medical blockade over at least 2 weeks allows depletion of catecholamine stores and restoration of intravascular volume.

Combined blockade with an alpha-adrenergic blocker (phenoxybenzamine) and a catecholamine synthesis inhibitor (metyrosine) generally results in patients that are well blocked and very responsive to pharmacological management during surgery.[6]

Calcium Channel Blockade

Calcium channel blockers have also been used to control blood pressure before and during pheochromocytoma surgery secondary to their relaxing effect on vascular smooth muscle.[7] Nifedipine (30–60 mg/day) has resulted in good pre-operative control of blood pressure. Vigorous intravenous hydration before surgery is used to restore intravascular volume. Theoretical advantages of calcium channel blockers include less orthostatic hypotension and better cardiac protection than that achieved with other regimens.

Intraoperative Management

The large sudden changes in blood pressure, and constricted total blood volume found in patients with pheochromocytoma, necessitate continuous monitoring of arterial blood pressure and the use of large-bore intravenous cannulae for volume replacement. Monitoring of arterial blood pressure should be instituted prior to intubation to recognize and treat significant and sudden blood pressure changes that can occur with this maneuver. Patients are sedated for arterial catheter placement, followed by induction of general anesthesia and placement of other vascular access, urethral catheterization, and intubation.

Anesthesia is induced using a sedative-hypnotic in combination with opioids and non-depolarizing neuromuscular blockade. Anesthetic agents causing histamine release are avoided. Anesthesia is maintained using an inhalational agent, avoiding halothane because of the resulting sensitization of the myocardium to catecholamines. Nitrous oxide can be used also to decrease inhalational agent requirements, although it is often avoided for laparoscopic procedures due to its propensity to collect in and distend the bowel. A central line placed after intubation is used to monitor central venous pressure and to administer vasoactive medications. A pulmonary arterial catheter may be useful in patients with cardiomyopathy or for other indications. Epidural catheters are commonly placed preoperatively for postoperative analgesia in patients scheduled to undergo open adrenalectomy.

Early ligation of the veins draining the tumor and avoidance of tumor manipulation will minimize the release of catecholamines into the circulation, although modern methods of blockade have made this less critical. Paroxysmal elevations in blood pressure are managed with phentolamine or nitroprusside. Tachycardias and tachydysrhythmias are treated with intravenous beta-blockers (e.g., esmolol, labetalol, lopressor, propanolol). Ligation of the main veins draining the tumor can result in severe hypotension, best treated with intravascular volume replacement with crystalloid. Short-term use of phenylephrine or norepinephrine may be required to support blood pressure as crystalloid is administered. The effectiveness of alpha-adrenergic agonists can be blunted due to the preoperative blockade.

Elevated levels of plasma catecholamines stimulate insulin production and lead to hyperglycemia. Removal of the tumor can be associated with hypoglycemia. Monitoring of glucose levels is performed during and after surgery until normal physiologic responses return.

LAPAROSCOPIC SURGERY

Choice of surgical approach is determined by the comfort of the surgeon with the use of laparoscopic surgery.[8–10] Laparoscopic removal of adrenal and extra-adrenal pheochromocytoma has been associated with more rapid recovery, lower narcotic use, shorter hospitalization, and fewer complications compared to those occurring with open surgery (reviewed in Smith et al.[10]). No tumor-size threshold has been identified as too large for laparoscopic surgery; hand-assisted laparoscopy has been used to remove pheochromocytomas as large as 15 cm. A relative indication for an open operation would include hemorrhage into tumor or a tumor in the renal hilum. Large hemorrhagic tumors can be friable and predisposed to rupture resulting in tumor spillage. Hilar tumors can become intimately involved with the renal vasculature and difficult to separate safely.

Surgery

Modern imaging techniques and biochemical blockade have supplanted the need for extensive abdominal exploration as part of pheochromocytoma surgery. These advances have contributed to laparoscopic excision of adrenal and extra-adrenal pheochromocytomas' rapidly becoming the standard of care. Laparoscopic and open surgery were found to have similar hemodynamic changes, need for intraoperative antihypertensive treatment during surgery, operative time, blood loss, and transfusion rate. Operative mortality has ranged from 0–2.3%.[11–16]

Postoperative Care

Patients are predisposed to orthostatic or resting hypotension after removal of the tumor due to the contracted intravascular volume associated with pheochromocytoma and the preoperative alpha blockade. Restoration of intravascular volume will correct the blood pressure while the effects of the blockade wear off (phenoxybenzamine, half-life of 24 hours; metyrosine, half-life of 4 hours). Hypertension can result from too vigorous repletion of intravascular volume or inadequately treated postoperative pain.

Follow-up Study

Catecholamine levels are evaluated about 6 weeks after the patient's discharge from the hospital to confirm removal of the pheochromocytoma. Persistent catecholamine excess can be associated with persistent multifocal or metastatic pheochromocytoma. Five-year survival after surgery has been 84–96%. Residual nonparoxysmal hypertension has been reported in 27 to 38% of patients after removal of pheochromocytoma and is attributed to essential hypertension. Tumor recurrence in patients with noninherited pheochromocytoma has been reported as 2% at 10 years, 7% at 15 years, and 9% at greater than 20 years after surgery.[14,17] Patients undergo yearly follow-up for recurrence of symptoms or hypertension and evaluation of catecholamines.

HEREDITARY FORMS OF PHEOCHROMOCYTOMA

About 10% of cases of pheochromocytoma are thought to occur related to an inherited genetic disorder, although incidence data would suggest a higher contribution. Hereditary forms of pheochromocytoma include von Hippel–Lindau disease (VHL), multiple endocrine neoplasia type 2 (MEN2), von Recklinghausen's neurofibromatosis, hereditary paraganglioma syndrome (PGL), and other poorly characterized forms of hereditary pheochromocytoma. All these hereditary forms of pheochromocytoma are inherited in an autosomal dominant fashion, although there is a variable penetrance.

Management of patients with hereditary forms of pheochromocytoma has included observation of small nonfunctional tumors and unilateral adrenalectomy for functional tumors. Prophylactic bilateral adrenalectomy has also been performed, but may not be curative as extra-adrenal tumors can also occur. Medical replacement therapy in these patients has resulted in a decreased quality of life. Twenty-five to 33% of patients on medical adrenal replacement have been reported to develop Addisonian crisis, which can rarely result in death.[18–20] After bilateral adrenalectomy, 30% of patients develop significant fatigue and 48% consider themselves handicapped.[19] Partial adrenalectomy, preserving adrenocortical function, can avoid the morbidity associated with medical adrenal replacement.[21,22]

Genetic Types

Von Hippel–Lindau Disease

Von Hippel–Lindau disease (VHL) is caused by inactivating mutations in the VHL gene, a tumor-suppressor gene (chromosome 3p25). VHL is characterized clinically by CNS hemangioblastoma, endolymphatic sac tumors, retinal angiomas, renal cysts and carcinomas, neuroendocrine tumors, cystadenoma, and simple cysts of the pancreas, epididymal cystadenomas, and/or pheochromocytoma, with variable presentation of each tumor type. VHL has been estimated to affect 1 in 36,000 persons.[23]

Only 16% of VHL pheochromocytomas have been reported to have related signs or symptoms. Affected VHL patients identified by screening present at an earlier age with fewer symptoms, less hypertension, lower urinary catecholamine excretion rates, and smaller tumors than do sporadic pheochromocytoma patients.[24] The primary catecholamine produced by VHL pheochromocytoma is norepinephrine. Twelve percent of VHL tumors have been reported to be extra-adrenal and 1.6% are associated with metastases. Missense mutations in the VHL gene have been most frequently associated with the development of pheochromocytoma in these families. In families with missense mutations, pheochromocytomas develop at a younger age, and extra-adrenal tumors and metastatic disease develop more frequently than is the case with families with other VHL gene mutation types.[24] It is noteworthy that VHL patients with pheochromocytoma identified by screening, as a group, have fewer functional tumors do than patients with sporadic tumors.

Multiple Endocrine Neoplasia Type 2

MEN2 is caused by activating mutations in the RET proto-oncogene (chromosome 10q11). MEN2A is characterized clinically by medullary thyroid cancer, parathyroid hyperplasia, and pheochromocytoma.[25] There is variable presentation of each tumor type. Patients with MEN2B, a less common variation, also develop mucosal ganglioneuromas. A germline mutation in codon 634 has been reported in 85% of MEN2A families.[26-28] The incidence of MEN2 has been estimated as 1 in 30,000 persons.

Pheochromocytomas in MEN2 patients are usually associated with elevated catecholamine excretion at first diagnosis, although about half of affected patients are asymptomatic and only a third hypertensive.[29] Both norepinephrine and epinephrine are produced by MEN2 pheochromocytoma. Extra-adrenal tumors are uncommon and about 70% of patients have bilateral adrenal tumors.[30,31]

Von Recklinghausen's Neurofibromatosis

Neurofibromatosis type 1 (NF-1) is caused by mutations in the NF-1 gene located on chromosome 17q11.[32] Patients with NF-1 develop neurofibromas and café-au-lait spots, and osseous lesions with a low penetrance of pheochromocytoma (0.1 to 5.7%) and carcinoid tumors. NF-1 is thought to affect about 1 in 3000 persons. About 40% of affected patients have no associated symptoms or hypertension. These patients with pheochromocytoma develop elevations in both epinephrine and norepinephrine excretion. Bilateral adrenal tumors (9.6%), extra-adrenal tumors (6.1%), and metastases (12%) are uncommon.

Hereditary Paraganglioma Syndrome (PGL1)

Hereditary paraganglioma syndrome is caused by mutations in the PGL1 gene, located on chromosome 11q23. Genomic imprinting occurs in hereditary paraganglioma syndrome; an autosomal dominant inheritance pattern is found in children of affected men, while children of affected women rarely develop the disease.[33] Patients present clinically with paragangliomas of the head and neck region (glomus tumors or chemodectomas, carotid body tumors).[33] About two-thirds of patients develop multiple tumors. About one in 100,000 persons are affected with hereditary paraganglioma syndrome.[33] Paraganglia in these patients may be nonfunctional.[34,35] Long-term remission has been associated with radiation treatment in a number of patients.[36,37]

Poorly Characterized Hereditary Pheochromocytoma

A few families have been reported with multiple members affected with pheochromocytoma, but no VHL or RET germline mutation.[38] Missense mutations of the VHL gene have been reported to be associated with pheochromocytoma and only subtle retinal angiomas or central nervous system hemangioblastomas.[39] Pheochromocytoma as the only manifestation of MEN2 has been poorly characterized in the literature.

Clinical Management

Diagnosis

At least 50 million Americans have or are treated for high blood pressure.[40] Patients selected for evaluation for sporadic pheochromocytoma generally have sudden-onset or malignant hypertension, tachycardia, tremor, sweating, poor response to standard medical therapy or are young in age. Twenty-four urinary excretion of catecholamines and plasma catecholamines are generally sufficient to confirm the diagnosis.[41] More recently, the use of plasma free metanephrines has proved to be a more sensitive and cost effective test.[42]

Familial forms of pheochromocytoma are identified by family history. Screening asymptomatic affected family members often identifies patients with small nonfunctional tumors. Patients with small hereditary pheochromocytomas are observed until tumors are functional as measured by urinary catecholamine excretion (greater than two times the upper limit of normal).[24] Although these patients often have elevated plasma free metanephrines, confirming the diagnosis, surgery can be safely delayed.

Periodic screening recommendations for familial pheochromocytoma vary in these diseases, based on tumor penetrance and typical age of presentation. Screening is routinely performed in these patients before any surgery or pregnancy is contemplated, or if symptoms do occur. Surgery has been recommended in these patients with localized tumors when catecholamine secretion became elevated, associated signs or symptoms occur, or when tumor size approaches 3 cm in diameter.

Observation of Tumors

Natural History of VHL Pheochromocytoma

Twelve VHL patients with no signs or symptoms of pheochromocytoma had 17 adrenal masses followed for a median of 35 months with no morbidity.[24] Patients with tumors were followed until urinary catecholamines became elevated more than two times the upper limit of normal. Median tumor doubling time was 17 months. Four of 12 patients developed functional pheochromocytoma within 23 months. Of the eight remaining patients, three developed MIBG uptake, plasma catecholamine, or provocative testing demonstrating function during follow-up. All tumors were less than 3.5 cm in diameter.

Laparoscopic Partial Adrenalectomy

Adrenocortical function has been preserved by means of partial adrenalectomy. Laparoscopic partial adrenalectomy has been shown to provide similar clinical results as open surgical partial adrenalectomy, with less surgical morbidity.[43–46] Small adrenal pheochromocytomas may not be visible and laparoscopic ultrasound can be required to localize a tumor. Precise localization allows limited mobilization of the normal adrenal gland and preservation of its vasculature. The right adrenal tail contains little or no medullary tissue,[47] and risk of recurrent adrenal pheochromocytoma in this location may be small. Clinical experience suggests that half to a third of one adrenal gland is sufficient to avoid adrenal medical replacement.

Partial adrenalectomy has been performed more frequently in small adrenal tumors (2.3 cm in diameter). Larger adrenal tumors (larger than 4 cm in diameter) result in greater distortion of the adrenal gland, making adrenocortical sparing techniques more difficult. Occasionally larger adrenal tumors located at one end of the adrenal gland can be resected with preservation of normal adrenal tissue. A frozen section can be helpful in these procedures as the margins are often small.

Patients are observed after partial adrenalectomy. If blood pressure is not easily maintained with fluid replacement, replacement doses of hydrocortisone are given to the patients until adrenocortical function can be assessed.[48]

Tumor Recurrence

Pheochromocytomas develop in the remaining adrenal gland in 19 to 33% of VHL patients a median of 4 years after unilateral adrenalectomy for pheochromocytoma.[24] Similarly, new pheochromocytomas developed in 52% of MEN2 patients a mean of 11.9 years after contralateral adrenalectomy.[20]

Patients undergoing partial adrenalectomy preserve adrenal cortical function, but also remain at risk for recurrent adrenal pheochromocytoma. As many as 20% of VHL patients have developed new pheochromocytoma a median of 40 months after partial adrenalectomy.[24] Similarly, MEN2 patients had a 0–33% risk of new pheochromocytoma during 54–88 months of follow-up.[49,50] No complications or metastases from recurrent pheochromocytoma have been reported in VHL or MEN2 patients undergoing partial adrenalectomy.[20–22,49]

Adrenal Medical Replacement

Standard medical adrenal replacement has consisted of glucocorticoid and mineralocorticoid replacement, and has been associated with normal longevity. In spite of this great medical advance, many patients complain of easy physical and mental fatigue, depression, and decreased libido. Women seem to be more frequently affected with these complaints. Postmenopausal women also seem to be predisposed to develop osteoporosis, a finding that has been linked to a decrease in circulating dehydroepiandrosterone (DHEA) levels.[51]

DHEA and its sulfated ester are normally produced in high amounts by the adrenal cortex, and levels decrease after menopause. Bilateral adrenalectomy removes the main source of this weak androgen, although some production occurs in the testicle, possible explaining a protective affect in men.[52]

In a randomized blinded study, the use of physiologic doses of DHEA in women (50 mg every morning) with adrenal insufficiency resulted in significant improvement in well-being and sexuality, compared to placebo.[53] Other studies have shown an improvement in bone parameters in postmenopausal women.[54] This developing evidence suggests that DHEA should be added as a third component of medical adrenal replacement.

ACKNOWLEDGMENTS

I extend special thanks to Graeme Eisenhofer and Hugh Preas for review and thoughtful comments.

REFERENCES

1. ANDERSEN, G.S., J.O. LUND, D. TOFTDAHL, *et al.* 1986. Pheochromocytoma and Conn's syndrome in Denmark 1977–1981. Acta Med. Scand. Suppl. **714:** 11–14.
2. HARTLEY, L. & D. PERRY-KEENE. 1985. Phaeochromocytoma in Queensland—1970–83. Aust. N. Z. J. Surg. **55:** 471–475.
3. STENSTROM, G. & K. SVARDSUDD. 1986. Pheochromocytoma in Sweden 1958—1981: an analysis of the National Cancer Registry Data. Acta Med. Scand. **220:** 225–232.
4. PERRY, R.R., H.R. KEISER, J.A. NORTON, *et al.* 1990. Surgical management of pheochromocytoma with the use of metyrosine. Ann. Surg. **212:** 621–628.
5. STEINSAPIR, J., A.A. CAR, L.M. PRISANT & E.D.J. BRANSOME. 1997. Metyrosine and pheochromocytoma. Arch. Intern. Med. **157:** 901–906.
6. VARGAS, H.I,. L.R. KAVOUSSI, D.L. BARTLETT, *et al.* 1997. Laparoscopic adrenalectomy: a new standard of care. Urology **49:** 673–678.
7. PROYE, C., D. THEVENIN, P. CECAT, *et al.* 1989. Exclusive use of calcium channel blockers in preoperative and intraoperative control of pheochromocytomas: hemodynamics and free catecholamine assays in ten consecutive patients. Surgery **106:** 1149–1154.

8. SPRUNG, J., J.F.J. O'HARA, I.S. GILL, et al. 2000. Anesthetic aspects of laparoscopic and open adrenalectomy for pheochromocytoma. Urology **55**: 339–343.
9. INABNET, W.B., J. PITRE, D. BERNARD & Y. CHAPUIS. 2000. Comparison of the hemodynamic parameters of open and laparoscopic adrenalectomy for pheochromocytoma. World J. Surg. **24**: 574–578.
10. SMITH, C.D., C.J. WEBER & J.R. AMERSON. 1999. Laparoscopic adrenalectomy: new gold standard. World J.Surg. **23**: 389–396.
11. OBARA, T., M. KANBE, T. OKAMOTO, et al. 1995. Surgical strategy for pheochromocytoma: emphasis on the pledge of flank extraperitoneal approach in selected patients. Surgery **118**: 1083–1089.
12. NAGESSER, S.K., J. KIEVIT, J. HERMANS, et al. 2000. The surgical approach to the adrenal gland: a comparison of the retroperitoneal and the transabdominal routes in 326 operations on 284 patients. Jpn. J. Clin. Oncol. **30**: 68–74.
13. GOLDSTEIN, R.E., J.A.J. O'NEILL, G.W. HOLCOMB, et al. 1999. Clinical experience over 48 years with pheochromocytoma. Ann. Surg. **229**: 755–764.
14. FAVIA, G., F. LUMACHI, F. POLISTINA & D.F. D'AMICO. 1998. Pheochromocytoma, a rare cause of hypertension: long-term follow-up of 55 surgically treated patients. World J.Surg. **22**: 689–693.
15. LUCON, A.M., M.A. PEREIRA, B.B. MENDONCA, et al. 1997. Pheochromocytoma: study of 50 cases. J. Urol. **157**: 1208–1212.
16. DUH, Q.Y. 2001. Evolving surgical management for patients with pheochromocytoma. J. Clin. Endocrinol. Metab. **86**: 1477–1479.
17. VAN HEERDEN, J.A., C.F. ROLAND, J.A. CARNEY, et al. 1990. Long-term evaluation following resection of apparently benign pheochromocytoma(s)/paraganglioma(s). World J. Surg. **14**: 325–329.
18. DE GRAAF, J.S., R.P. DULLAART & R.P. ZWIERSTRA. 1999. Complications after bilateral adrenalectomy for phaeochromocytoma in multiple endocrine neoplasia type 2: a plea to conserve adrenal function. Eur. J. Surg. **165**: 843–846.
19. TELENIUS-BERG, M., M.A. PONDER, B. BERG, et al. 1989. Quality of life after bilateral adrenalectomy in MEN 2. Henry Ford Hosp. Med. J. **37**: 160–163.
20. LAIRMORE, T.C., D.W. BALL, S.B. BAYLIN & S.A. WELLS, JR. 1993. Management of pheochromocytomas in patients with multiple endocrine neoplasia type 2 syndromes. Ann. Surg. **217**: 595–603.
21. WALTHER, M.M., H.R. KEISER, P.L. CHOYKE, et al. 1999. Management of hereditary pheochromocytoma in Von Hippel Lindau kindreds with partial adrenalectomy. J. Urol. **161**: 395–398.
22. LEE, J.E., S.A. CURLEY, R.F. GAGEL, et al. 1996. Cortical-sparing adrenalectomy for patients with bilateral pheochromocytoma. Surgery **120**: 1064–1070.
23. LINEHAN, W.M., M.I. LERMAN & B. ZBAR. 1995. Identification of the von Hippel-Lindau (VHL) gene: its role in renal cancer. JAMA **273**: 564–570.
24. WALTHER, M,M., R. REITER, H.R. KEISER, et al. Clinical and genetic characterization of pheochromocytoma in Von Hippel-Lindau families: comparison with sporadic pheochromocytoma gives insight into natural history of pheochromocytoma. J. Urol. **162**: 659–664.
25. LIPS, C.J., R.M. LANDSVATER, J.W. HOPPENER, et al. 1994. Clinical screening as compared with DNA analysis in families with multiple endocrine neoplasia type 2A. N. Engl. J. Med. **331**: 828–835.

26. EGAWA, S., H. FUTAMI, K. TAKASAKI, et al. 1998. Genotype-phenotype correlation of patients with multiple endocrine neoplasia type 2 in Japan. Jpn. J. Clin. Oncol. **28:** 590–596.
27. ENG, C., D. CLAYTON, I. SCHUFFENECKER, et al. 1996. The relationship between specific RET proto-oncogene mutations and disease phenotype in multiple endocrine neoplasia type 2. International RET mutation consortium analysis. JAMA **276:** 1575–1579.
28. RAUE, F. 1998. German medullary thyroid carcinoma/multiple endocrine neoplasia registry: German MTC/MEN Study Group—medullary thyroid carcinoma/multiple endocrine neoplasia type 2. Langenbecks Arch. Surg. **383:** 334–336.
29. POMARES, F.J., R. CANAS, J.M. RODRIGUEZ, et al. 1998. Differences between sporadic and multiple endocrine neoplasia type 2A phaeochromocytoma. Clin. Endocrinol. (Oxford). **48:** 195–200.
30. LIPS, C.J., R.M. LANDSVATER, J.W. HOPPENER, et al. 1995. From medical history and biochemical tests to presymptomatic treatment in a large MEN 2A family. J. Intern. Med. **238:** 347–356.
31. NEUMANN, H.P., D.P. BERGER, G. SIGMUND, et al. 1993. Pheochromocytomas, multiple endocrine neoplasia type 2, and von Hippel-Lindau disease. N. Engl. J. Med. **329:** 1531–1538.
32. WALTHER, M.M., J. HERRING, E. ENQUIST, et al. 1999. von Recklinghausen's disease and pheochromocytomas. J. Urol. **162:** 1582–1586.
33. VAN SCHOTHORST, E.M., J.C. JANSEN, A.F. BARDOEL, et al. 1996. Confinement of PGL, an imprinted gene causing hereditary paragangliomas, to a 2-cM interval on 11q22-q23 and exclusion of DRD2 and NCAM as candidate genes. Eur. J. Hum. Genet. **4:** 267–273.
34. PARKIN, J.L. 1981. Familial multiple glomus tumors and pheochromocytomas. Ann.Otol. Rhinol. Laryngol. **90:** 60–63.
35. MCCAFFREY, T.V., F.B. MEYER, V.V. MICHELS, et al. 1994. Familial paragangliomas of the head and neck. Arch. Otolaryngol. Head. Neck Surg. **120:** 1211–1216.
36. POWELL, S., N. PETERS & C. HARMER. 1992. Chemodectoma of the head and neck: results of treatment in 84 patients. Int. J. Radiat. Oncol. Biol. Phys. **22:** 919–924.
37. SKOLYSZEWSKI, J., S. KORZENIOWSKI & J. PSZON. 1991. Results of radiotherapy in chemodectoma of the temporal bone. Acta Oncol. **30:** 847–849.
38. SKOLDBERG, F., L. GRIMELIUS, E.R. WOODWARD, et al. 1998. A family with hereditary extra-adrenal paragangliomas without evidence for mutations in the von Hippel-Lindau disease or ret genes. Clin. Endocrinol.(Oxford) **48:** 11–16.
39. RITTER, M.M., A. FRILLING, P.A. CROSSEY, et al. 1996. Isolated familial pheochromocytoma as a variant of von Hippel-Lindau disease. J. Clin. Endocrinol. Metab. **81:** 1035–1037.
40. NAKAJO, M., B. SHAPIRO, J. COPP, et al. 1983. The normal and abnormal distribution of the adrenomedullary imaging agent m-[I-131]iodobenzylguanidine (I-131 MIBG) in man: evaluation by scintigraphy. J. Nucl. Med. **24:** 672–682.
41. BRAVO, E.L. 1991. Diagnosis of pheochromocytoma: reflections on a controversy. Hypertension **17:** 742–744.
42. LENDERS, J.W., H.R. KEISE, D.S. GOLDSTEIN, et al. 1995. Plasma metanephrines in the diagnosis of pheochromocytoma. Ann. Intern. Med. **123:** 101–109.

43. PULLERITS, J., S. EIN & J.W. BALFE. 1988. Anaesthesia for phaeochromocytoma. Can. J. Anaesth. **35:** 526–534.
44. WALTHER, M.M., J. HERRING, P.L. CHOYKE & W.M. LINEHAN. 2000. Laparoscopic partial adrenalectomy in patients with hereditary forms of pheochromocytoma. J. Urol. In press.
45. NEUMANN, H.P., M. REINCKE, B.U. BENDER, et al. 1999. Preserved adrenocortical function after laparoscopic bilateral adrenal sparing surgery for hereditary pheochromocytoma. J. Clin. Endocrinol. Metab. **84:** 2608–2610.
46. GILL, I.S. 2001. The case for laparoscopic adrenalectomy. J. Urol.. **166:** 429–436.
47. DOBBIE, J.W. & T. SYMINGTON. 1966. The human adrenal gland with special reference to the vasculature. J. Endocrin. **34:** 479–489.
48. DOHERTY, G.M., L.K. NIEMAN, G.B. CUTLE, JR., et al. 1990. Time to recovery of the hypothalamic-pituitary-adrenal axis after curative resection of adrenal tumors in patients with Cushing's syndrome. Surgery **108:** 1085–1090.
49. ALBANESE, C.T. & E.S. WIENER. 1993. Routine total bilateral adrenalectomy is not warranted in childhood familial pheochromocytoma. J. Pediatr. Surg. **28:** 1248–1252.
50. OKAMOTO, T., T. OBARA, Y. ITO, et al. 1996. Bilateral adrenalectomy with autotransplantation of adrenocortical tissue or unilateral adrenalectomy: treatment options for pheochromocytomas in multiple endocrine neoplasia type 2A. Endocr. J. **43:** 169–175.
51. DEVOGELAER, J.P., J. CRABBE & D.D. NAGANT. 1987. Bone mineral density in Addison's disease. Br. Med. J. (Clin. Res. Ed.) **295:** 214
52. KROBOTH, P.D., F.S. SALEK, A.L. PITTENGER, et al. 1999. DHEA and DHEA-S: a review. J. Clin. Pharmacol. **39:** 327–348.
53. ARLT, W., F. CALLIES, J.C. VAN VLIJMEN, et al. 1999. Dehydroepiandrosterone replacement in women with adrenal insufficiency. N. Engl. J. Med. **341:** 1013–1020.
54. BAULIEU, E.E., G. THOMAS, S. LEGRAIN, et al. 2000. Dehydroepiandrosterone (DHEA), DHEA sulfate, and aging: contribution of the DHEAge Study to a sociobiomedical issue. Proc. Natl. Acad. Sci. USA. **97:** 4279–4284.

Radiopharmaceutical Treatment of Pheochromocytomas

JAMES C. SISSON

University of Michigan Health System, Ann Arbor, Michigan 48109-0028, USA

ABSTRACT: Malignant pheochromocytomas, a group of tumors that include metastatic paragangliomas, often produce hypertension and episodic symptoms from secretion of norepinephrine and sometimes epinephrine. In addition, the tumors usually manifest progressive metastases. Blockade of alpha and beta adrenergic receptors will control blood pressure and symptoms, but reduction of the malignancy has been difficult to achieve. Meta-iodobenzylguanidine (MIBG) follows the pathways of norepinephrine and, when labeled with 131-I, will concentrate sufficiently in the pheochromocytoma to impart therapeutic radiation. More than 100 patients have received treatment with 131-I-labeled MIBG at multiple medical centers. Individual doses were 3.7 to 18.5 GBq (100 to >500 mCi), and many patients received several doses separated by a few months. Partial remissions, recorded as decreased tumor presence and tumor function, have been observed in one-third or more of the treated patients. However, complete remissions are rare, and recurrence/progression within two years is the rule. Toxicity was generally modest and temporary. Subsequent chemotherapy increased the benefits attained by 131-I MIBG, but, in a small series of patients, this combination did not further change the outcome. Nevertheless, selective radiation from 131-I MIBG or a similar radiopharmaceutical could play a valuable role in treatments that combine several types of attacks on this recalcitrant malignancy.

KEYWORDS: pheochromocytoma; paraganglioma; malignancy; meta-iodobenzylguanidine

INTRODUCTION

Although pheochromocytomas are rare neoplasms and constitute only about 0.1% of the causes of hypertension,[1] these tumors derive importance from the sometimes dramatic clinical presentations resulting from secreted neurohormones, and by often being cured by surgical excision. Included in

---

Address for correspondence: James C. Sisson, M.D., Hospital B1 505G, University of Michigan Health System, Ann Arbor, MI 48109-0028. Voice: 734-936-5387; fax: 734-936-8182.
jsisson@umich.edu

the category of pheochromocytomas are the paragangliomas, those tumors with the same potentials but arising from adrenergic tissues outside of the adrenal medulla.

About 10–15% of pheochromocytomas are metastatic,[2] and, because of anatomic dispersal, cannot be fully resected. For these carcinomas, therapy beyond surgical excision must be sought. Pharmacologic blockade of alpha and beta adrenergic receptors will usually relieve the hypertension and symptoms arising from the effects of the neurohormones, norepinephrine and epinephrine, but do not impede neoplastic growth. Chemotherapy, consisting of cylophosphamide, dacarbazine and vincristine, has produced one complete and several partial remissions[3]; however, the program requires considerable skill and time to administer and is not well-tolerated by some patients. External beam radiation can lessen pain caused by individual tumors, but the courses of malignant pheochromocytomas are unaltered. The radiopharmaceutical, 131-I-labeled meta-iodobenzylguanidine (131-I-MIBG), was found, during diagnostic study, to concentrate in about 85–90% of pheochromocytomas, including metastases.[4] From quantified scintigraphic data, the potential for delivering selective radiation to the unresectable tumors was recognized.[5]

Although classified as an analogue of guanethidine, MIBG (FIG. 1) follows the kinetic pathways of norepinephrine. 131-I-labled MIBG enters adrenergic cells via the uptake-1 pathway and is sequestered by the storage granules.[6] It is released from the cells by exocytosis[7] and, to some extent, by reversal of the uptake pathway. The agent appears not to bind to adrenergic receptors and thus has no direct pharmacologic action[8]; however, in large quantities, it may exhibit a tyramine-like effect by displacing norepinephrine from nerve terminals.[7] When concentrated and retained in substantial amounts by the tumors, the radiation imparted by the 131-I label can be therapeutic. About 90% of the radiation will be derived from the beta particle, from which most of the energy is deposited along a path of 1 mm. Thus, the radiation from 131-I MIBG is largely confined to targeted pheochromocytomas. The common therapeutic prescriptions have been 3.7–7.4 GBq (100–200 mCi).[9] A concentration of 131-I MIBG of 0.1% of the administered radioactivity per gram of tumor and an effective half life in the tumor of 3 days were reasonable estimates from diagnostic data of some patients; in this circumstance administration of 100 mCi to a patient will impart 4000–5000 cGy (rad) to the pheochromocytomas. Measurements recorded 13–82 cGy/mCi for tumors in a number of patients,[10] and >5000 cGy can be attained with multiple treatments in selected patients.[11] The radiopharmaceutical is also concentrated in normal adrenergic tissues, particularly neuron terminals and the adrenal medulla, but therapeutic doses of 131-I MIBG have not produced observable changes in these organs. The serious toxic effects have been largely confined to depression of bone marrow function.

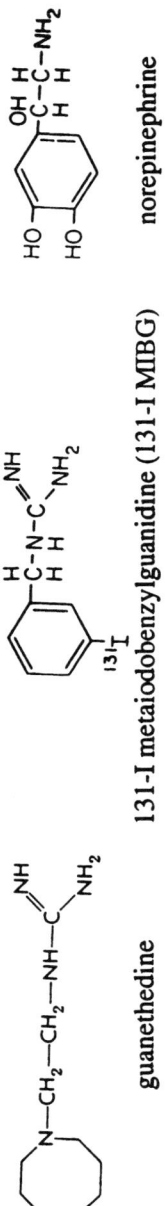

FIGURE 1. Molecular structures for comparisons.

TABLE 1. Results of treatment of pheochromocytoma with 131-I-labeled MIBG

	No. of patients	Complete remission[a] (%)	Partial remission[a] (%)	Little or no change (%)	Progression of disease (%)
Literature review[9]					
Tumor presence[a]	116	4	26	57	13
Tumor function[a]	96	13	32	45	10
Literature review[12]					
Tumor presence[a]	137	6	18	55	21
Tumor function[a]	120		39[b]		
University of Michigan[c]					
Tumor presence[a]	6	0	33	33	33
Tumor function[a]	6	17	17	33	33

[a]See text for definitions of remission and tumor presence and function.
[b]Includes partial and complete remission.
[c]Changes observed before chemotherapy was given.[11]

RESULTS FROM TREATMENTS WITH 131-I MIBG

In a review of the literature in 1997 (TABLE 1), Loh et al. found reports covering 116 patients treated for malignant/unresectable pheochromocytomas by 131-I MIBG; the authors added 3 patients of their own.[9] Most treatments were of 3.7–7.4 GBq that were given multiple times separated by several months to individual patients. A subsequent review by Troncone and Rufini in 1999[12] increased the total to 137 patients including 28 treated at the University of Michigan up to that time (TABLE 1).[10] In single infusions of 131-I MIBG, more than 11.1 GBq have been administered,[11] and one patient received more than 18.5 GBq.[9] Responses to the therapies were defined in terms of tumor presence (determined by CT, 131-I MIBG scintigraphy and/or bone scintigraphy) and tumor function (assayed by rates of urinary excretion of catecholamines and/or catecholamine metabolites). Some of the patients in the published papers did not have clearly defined tumor presence or function so that the numbers of patients in each index did not regularly equal the total number of patients treated.

Complete remissions (disappearance of all evidence of tumor presence and function) were uncommon, and some of those so classified exhibited small tumors seen only by MIBG scintigraphy[13–15] and/or had little or no elevations in the indices of tumor function.[9,15] Partial remissions (reduction of tumor presence and/or tumor function by half or more) occurred in 18–39% of patients giving complete plus partial remission rates of 24–45%. There was no obvious relationship between remission and administered dose. Relapses and/or progression of disease within two years were the rule.

Stable disease was reported for 33–60% of patients after treatment with 131-I MIBG. Although it is tempting to attribute stability to irradiation from 131-I MIBG, such carcinomas have often run indolent courses and, in the past, as many as 17% of patients have survived more than 20 years.[2]

Toxicity from 131-I MIBG was modest for most treated patients. Most vulnerable was the bone marrow; one patient died from pancytopenia.[16] Nausea and vomiting, at times severe for a few days, was common.[9–12] Liver dysfunction followed treatments of patients with liver metastases.[9] Exacerbation of manifestations of excessive catecholamines appeared in some subjects.[9,12] Hypothyroidism, presumably from thyroid sequestration of 131-I iodide metabolized from the 131-I MIBG, has occasionally occurred despite preventive treatments with stable iodides.[9,10,12]

Added to TABLE 1 are data from the latest experience with six patients at the University of Michigan.[11] Following three treatments with 131-I MIBG at 3-month intervals, there were partial remissions in tumor presence for two patients; one patient whose functional abnormality was modest had a complete remission and another had a partial remission in tumor function. Chemotherapy (cyclophosphamide, dacarbazine and vincristine in cycles over one year) was associated with further diminutions in tumor presence and function. However, toxicities—neutropenia, anemia and neuropathy—from the chemotherapy required reductions in doses of individual agents. In this small group of patients receiving these combined modalities, benefits from the additional chemotherapy were modest but demonstrated that attacks on malignant pheochromocytomas in multiple ways may be an effective approach to these resistant tumors.

DISCUSSION

131-I-labeled MIBG is selectively concentrated in many malignant pheochromocytomas to a level enabling therapeutic radiation of >5000 and possibly 20,000 cGy from multiple doses of this radiopharmaceutical. However, complete remissions have been rare, and the patients who have developed partial remissions in tumor presence and/or function usually exhibit relapses within 2 years. Probably the carcinomas consist of cells with varying affinities for 131-I MIBG, and, therefore the irradiation by 131-I is unevenly distributed within the tumors.

Although the initial experience with multiple-modality treatment (that is, adding a chemotherapy program to treatments with 131-I MIBG) did not demonstrate striking results, there was an additive effect. Possibly a third type of treatment, such as adding autologous bone marrow transplantation after higher doses of 131-I MIBG and more intensive chemotherapy, will produce better results.

SUMMARY

Malignant pheochromocytomas have resisted therapies. Selective irradiation from multiple doses of 131-I MIBG reduced tumor presence and function, resulting in remissions, partial and complete, in 24–45% of patients. Because most patients have unyielding tumors and because relapses are common in the responsive pheochromocytomas, additional treatments must be sought. Multi-modality therapies may improve the outcomes.

ACKNOWLEDGMENT

The author is indebted to Ms. Carol Kruise for help in typing.

REFERENCES

1. MANGER, W.M. & R.W. GIFFORD, JR. 1996. *In* Clinical and Experimental Pheochromocytoma, 2nd ed. W.M. Manger & R.W. Gifford, Jr. Eds.: 4. Blackwell Science, Inc. Cambridge, MA..
2. REMINE W.H., G.C. CHONG, J.A. VAN HEERDEN, et al. 1974. Current management of pheochromocytoma. Ann. Surg. **30:** 740–747.
3. AVERBUCH, S.D., C.S. STEAKLEY, R.C. YOUNG, et al. 1988. Malignant pheochromocytoma: effective treatment with a combination of cyclophosphamide, vincristine, and dacarbazine. Ann. Intern. Med. **109:** 267–273.
4. SHAPIRO, B., J.E. COPP, J.C. SISSON, et al. 1985. Iodine-131 metaiodobenzylguanidine for the locating of suspected pheochromocytoma: experience in 400 cases. J. Nucl. Med. **26:** 576–585.
5. SISSON, J.C., B. SHAPIRO, W.H. BEIERWALTES, et al. 1984. Radiopharmaceutical treatment of malignant pheochromocytoma. J. Nucl. Med. **25:** 197–206.
6. JAQUES, S., M.C. TOBES & J.C. SISSON. 1987. Sodium dependency of uptake of norepinephrine and m-iodobenzylguanidine into cultured human pheochromocytoma cells: evidence for uptake-one. Cancer Res. **47:** 3920–3928.
7. SISSON J.C., D.M. WEILAND, P. SHERMAN, et al. 1987 Metaiodobenzylguanidine as an index of the adrenergic nervous system intergrity and function. J. Nucl. Med. **28:** 1620–1624.
8. WIELAND, D.M., L.E. BROWN, M.C. TOBES, et al. 1981. Imagine the primate adrenal medullae with [^{123}I] and [^{131}I] meta-iodobenzylguanidine: concise communication. J. Nucl. Med. **22:** 358–364.
9. LOH, K.C., P.A. FITZGERALD, K.K. MATTHAY, et al. 1997. The treatment of malignant pheochromocytoma with iodine-131 metaiodobenzylguanidine

(131I-MIBG): a comprehensive review of 116 reported patients. J. Endocrinol.Invest. **20:** 648–658.
10. SHAPIRO, B., J.C. SISSON, D.M. WIELAND, *et al.* 1992. Radiopharmaceutical therapy of malignant pheochromocytoma with [^{131}I] metaiodobenzylguanidine: results from ten years of experience. J. Nucl. Biol. Med. **35:** 267–276.
11. SISSON J.C., B. SHAPIRO, B.S. SHULKIN, *et al.* 1999. Treatment of malignant pheochromocytomas with 131-I metaiodobenzylguanidine and chemotherapy. Am. J. Clin. Oncol. **22:** 364–370.
12. TRONCONE L. & V. RUFINI. 1999. Nuclear medicine therapy of pheochromocytoma and paraganglioma. Quart. J. Med. **43:** 344–355.
13. SCHVARTZ, C., C. GIBOLD, B. VUILLEMIN, *et al.* 1992. Results of [^{131}I] metaiodobenzylguanidine therapy administered to three patients with malignant pheochromocytoma. J. Nucl. Biol. Med. **35:** 305–307.
14. TRONCONE, L., V. RUFINI, P. MONTEMAGGI, *et al.* 1990. The diagnostic and therapeutic utility of radioiodinated metaiodobenzylguanidine. Eur. J. Nucl. Med. **16:** 325–335.
15. TRONCONE, L., V. RUFINI, M.S. DALDONE, *et al.* 1991. [^{131}I] metaiodobenzylguanidine treatment of malignant pheochromocytoma: experience of the Rome group. J. Nucl. Biol. Med. **35:** 295–299.
16. KREMPF, M., J. LUMBROSO, R. MOREX., *et al.* 1991. Use of m-[^{131}I] iodobenzylguanidine in the treatment of malignant pheochromocytoma. J. Clin. Endocrinol. Metab. **72:** 455–461.

Primary Aldosteronism
Management Issues

WILLIAM F. YOUNG, JR.

Division of Endocrinology and Metabolism, and Internal Medicine, Mayo Clinic and Mayo Foundation, Rochester, Minnesota 55905, USA

ABSTRACT: Since its initial description in 1955, primary aldosteronism was thought to be a rare cause of hypertension. However, improved screening methods show that primary aldosteronism is a common form of secondary hypertension. Diagnosis of this disorder results in improved or cured hypertension or targeted pharmacotherapy. Patients with hypertension and hypokalemia and most patients with treatment-resistant hypertension should undergo screening for primary aldosteronism. A random and ambulatory ratio of plasma aldosterone concentration (PAC) to plasma renin activity (PRA) that is elevated and a PAC higher than a set cutoff is a positive screen for primary aldosteronism. An increased PAC/PRA ratio alone is not diagnostic of primary aldosteronism; primary aldosteronism must be confirmed by demonstrating inappropriate aldosterone secretion with either the intravenous saline suppression test or measurement of 24-hr urinary aldosterone while the patient is on a high-sodium diet. The two major subtypes of primary aldosteronism are unilateral aldosterone-producing adenoma (APA) and bilateral idiopathic hyperplasia (IHA). Patients with APA are usually treated with unilateral adrenalectomy, and patients with IHA are treated medically. The subtype evaluation may require one or more tests, the first of which is imaging the adrenals with computerized tomography (CT). When a solitary unilateral macroadenoma (> 1 cm) and normal contralateral adrenal morphologic pattern are found on CT in a young patient with primary aldosteronism, unilateral laparoscopic adrenalectomy is a reasonable therapeutic option. However, in many cases, CT imaging may reveal normal-appearing adrenals or ambiguous findings. Adrenal venous sampling helps to resolve these clinical dilemmas.

KEYWORDS: hyperaldosteronism; hypertension; adrenal; hypokalemia

Address for correspondence: William F. Young, Jr., M.D., Mayo Clinic, W18 Mayo Building, 200 First Street S.W., Rochester, MN 55905. Voice: 507-284-2191; fax: 507-284-5745.
Young.William@Mayo.edu

INTRODUCTION

The syndrome of primary aldosteronism, first described in 1955, is characterized by hypertension, suppressed plasma renin activity (PRA), increased plasma aldosterone concentration (PAC), and unsuppressible aldosterone levels in the blood or urine.[1] Prevalence estimates for primary aldosteronism when hypokalemia was one of the diagnostic criteria varied from 0.05–2% of the population with hypertension. However, with improved screening methods and the recognition that most patients with primary aldosteronism are normokalemic, it appears that primary aldosteronism is the most common form of secondary hypertension.[2–5] Current prevalence estimates range from 5 to 10% of the hypertensive population.[2–5]

Distinguishing the subtype of primary aldosteronism is critical to appropriate therapy. Conn's first case was a 34-year-old woman with a 4-cm unilateral aldosterone-producing adenoma (APA). A more common subtype of primary aldosteronism is idiopathic hyperaldosteronism (IHA) due to bilateral zona glomerulosa hyperplasia (TABLE 1).[6,7] Primary adrenal hyperplasia (PAH), or unilateral adrenal hyperplasia, is an uncommon subtype. A hyperplastic adrenal that morphologically resembles that in IHA but mimics the APA response to physiologic maneuvers and unilateral or subtotal adrenalectomy characterizes PAH.[6,8] Glucocorticoid-remediable aldosteronism (GRA) is autosomal dominant in inheritance and is associated with variable degrees of hyperaldosteronism, high levels of hybrid steroids (e.g., 18-hydroxycortisol), and suppression with exogenous glucocorticoid.[9,10]

Unilateral adrenalectomy cures hypokalemia in all patients and improves or cures hypertension in most patients who have APA or PAH, whereas surgery is not as effective for patients with IHA or GRA. The key management issues in primary aldosteronism are screening, confirmatory testing, subtype evaluation, and treatment.

TABLE 1. Subtypes of primary aldosteronism

May be Treated Surgically for Cure:

    Aldosterone-producing adenoma (APA)

    Primary (unilateral) adrenal hyperplasia (PAH)

    Aldosterone-producing adrenocortical carcinoma

Should be Treated Medically:

    Idiopathic hyperaldosteronism (IHA)

    Glucocorticoid-remediable aldosteronism (GRA)

DIAGNOSIS

The diagnosis of primary aldosteronism is usually made in patients in the third to sixth decades. Few symptoms are specific to the syndrome. Patients with marked hypokalemia may have muscle weakness, cramping, headaches, palpitation, polydipsia, polyuria, or nocturia. There are no specific physical findings. The degree of hypertension is usually moderate to severe and may be resistant to usual pharmacologic treatments.[6,7] Hypokalemia is frequently absent, and thus all patients with hypertension are candidates for this disorder. Several studies have shown that patients with primary aldosteronism may be at higher risk than other hypertension patients for target organ damage of the heart and kidney.[11–17] Hypokalemia reduces the secretion of aldosterone and it is optimal to bring the serum potassium into the normal range before performing diagnostic studies.

Screening Tests

Spontaneous hypokalemia is uncommon in patients with uncomplicated hypertension and, when present, strongly suggests associated mineralocorticoid excess. However, normokalemia does not exclude primary aldosteronism. Several studies have shown that most patients with primary aldosteronism have baseline serum levels of potassium in the normal range.[2,18,19] Therefore, hypokalemia is not required to make the diagnosis of primary aldosteronism. Patients with hypertension and hypokalemia, regardless of presumed cause (e.g., diuretic treatment), and most patients with treatment-resistant hypertension should undergo screening for primary aldosteronism (FIG. 1).

Screening can be accomplished in patients with suspected primary aldosteronism by measuring a morning (preferably 8 AM) ambulatory paired random plasma aldosterone concentration (PAC) and PRA (FIG. 1). Usually PAC is measured in ng/dL and PRA is measured in ng/mL/hr. This test may be performed while the patient is on antihypertensive medications and without posture stimulation.[20] Spironolactone is the only known medication that will absolutely interfere with interpretation of the ratio. Angiotensin-converting enzyme (ACE) inhibitors have the potential to "falsely elevate" PRA. Therefore, in a patient treated with an ACE-inhibitor, the findings of a detectable PRA level or a low PAC/PRA ratio do not exclude the diagnosis of primary aldosteronism. In addition, a strong predictor for primary aldosteronism is a PRA level undetectably low in a patient taking an ACE-inhibitor.

The PAC/PRA ratio, first proposed as a screening test for primary aldosteronism in 1981,[21] is based on the concept of paired hormone measurements (FIG. 2).[22] For example, in the hypertensive hypokalemic patient: (1) secondary hyperaldosteronism should be considered when both PRA and PAC are

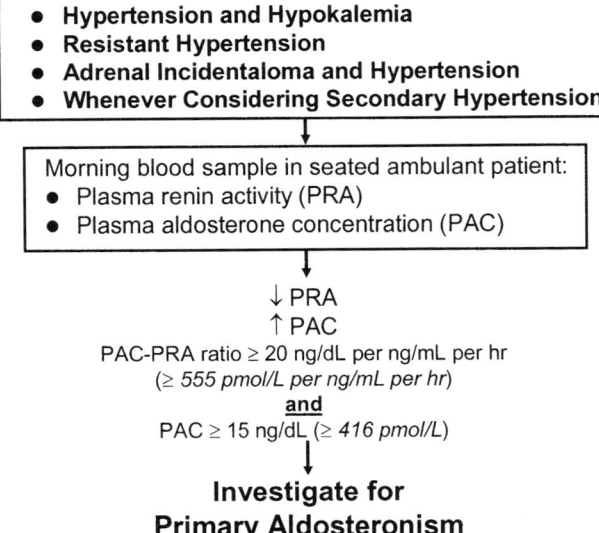

FIGURE 1. Use of the PAC/PRA ratio to screen for primary aldosteronism. PAC, plasma aldosterone concentration; PRA, plasma renin activity.

increased and the PAC/PRA ratio is < 10 (e.g., renovascular disease); (2) alternate source of mineralocorticoid receptor agonism should be considered when both PRA and PAC are suppressed (e.g., hypercortisolism); and (3) primary aldosteronism should be suspected when PRA is suppressed and PAC is increased (FIG. 3). Fourteen prospective studies have been published on use of the PAC/PRA ratio in screening for primary aldosteronism.[2,3,20,21,23–33] Although there is some uncertainty about test characteristics and lack of standardization,[34] the PAC/PRA is widely accepted as the screening test of choice for primary aldosteronism.[35,36] It has erroneously been suggested that the PAC/PRA ratio is not useful because is does not provide a renin-independent measure of circulating aldosterone that is suitable for determining whether PAC is elevated relative to PRA.[37] However, the diagnostic value of the PAC/PRA ratio is denominator-dependent (FIG. 2) and it is not an independent "index." A suppressed level of PRA is critical to the diagnosis of primary aldosteronism—just as a suppressed level of TSH is a key finding in hyperthyroidism.

It is important to understand that the lower limit of detection varies among the different PRA assays and can have a dramatic effect on the PAC/PRA ratio.[4,37,38] As an example, a very different ratio is obtained if the lower limit of detection for PRA is 0.6 ng/mL per hour compared to 0.1 ng/mL per hour;

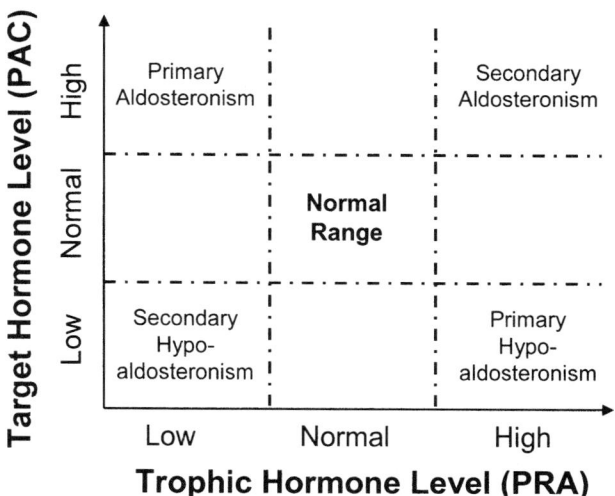

FIGURE 2. Paired hormone measurements help to differentiate among the different types of hyper- and hypofunction of the renin–angiotensin–aldosterone axis.

for a PAC of 16 ng/dL, the PAC/PRA ratio would be 27 and 160, respectively. Thus, the cutoff for a "high" PAC/PRA ratio is laboratory-dependent and, more specifically, PRA assay-dependent. In addition, a cutoff for PAC should be established to be used in conjuction with the PAC/PRA ratio. For example, Weinberger and colleagues found that the combination of a PAC/PRA ratio > 30 *and* PAC > 20 ng/dL had a sensitivity of 90% and a specificity of 91% for aldosterone-producing adenomas.[39] Hirohira and colleagues found that a PAC/PRA ratio of > 32 had a sensitivity of 100% and specificity of 61% for APA.[38] In our laboratory, we use a PAC (in ng/dL)/PRA (in ng/mL per hour) ratio ≥ 20 *and* PAC ≥ 15 ng/dL to indicate probable primary aldosteronism. A high PAC/PRA ratio and a PAC value in the mid-normal range or higher is a positive screening test result, a finding that warrants further testing.

Confirmatory Tests

An elevated PAC/PRA ratio is not diagnostic by itself, and primary aldosteronism must be confirmed by demonstrating inappropriate aldosterone secretion. The list of drugs and hormones capable of affecting the renin–angiotensin–aldosterone axis is extensive, and frequently in patients with severe hypertension, a "medication-contaminated" evaluation is unavoidable. Calcium channel blockers, α_1-adrenergic receptor blockers, and β-adrenergic receptor blockers do not affect the diagnostic accuracy in most cases.[40] It is impossible to interpret data obtained from patients receiving treatment with

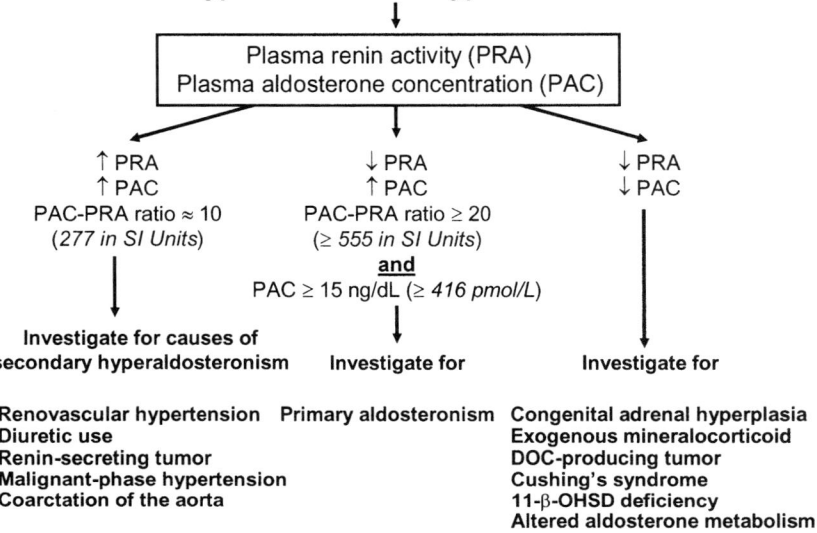

FIGURE 3. Use of the PAC/PRA ratio to differentiate among the different causes of hypertension and hypokalemia. PAC, plasma aldosterone concentration; PRA, plasma renin activity. (Modified from Young and Hogan[6] by permission.)

spironolactone. Therefore, spironolactone treatment should not be initiated until the evaluation is completed and the final decisions about treatment are made. If primary aldosteronism is suspected in a patient receiving treatment with spironolactone, the treatment should be discontinued for at least 6 weeks prior to testing.

Aldosterone suppression testing can be performed with orally administered sodium chloride and measurement of urinary aldosterone or with intravenous sodium chloride loading and measurement of PAC.[18,40,41] Our protocol uses oral salt loading over 3 days. After hypertension and hypokalemia are controlled, patients should receive a high-sodium diet (supplemented with sodium chloride tablets if needed) for 3 days. The risk of increasing dietary sodium in patients with severe hypertension must be assessed in each case. Because the high-salt diet can increase kaliuresis and hypokalemia, vigorous replacement of potassium chloride may be needed and serum potassium should be monitored daily. On the third day of the high-sodium diet, a 24-hour urine specimen is collected for measurement of aldosterone, sodium, and potassium. The 24-hour urinary sodium excretion should exceed 200 mEq to document adequate sodium repletion. Urinary aldosterone excretion >12 μg/24 hours in this setting is consistent with autonomous aldosterone secretion.[42]

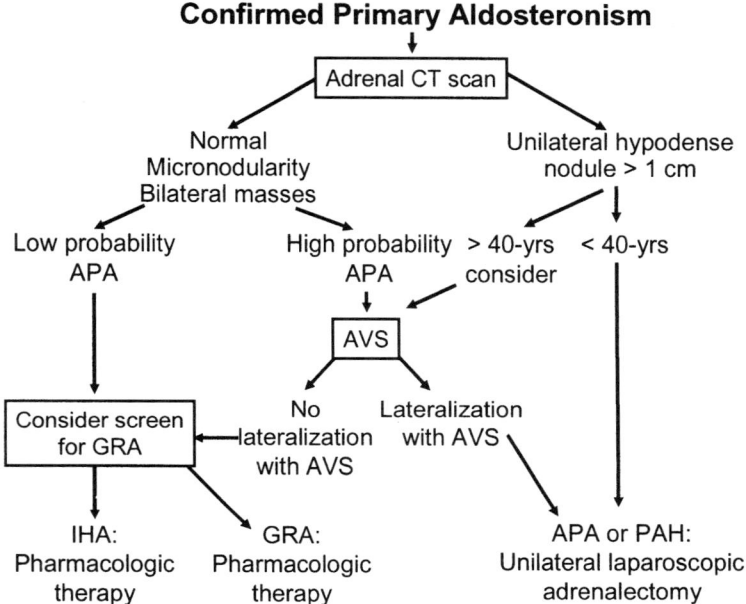

FIGURE 4. Subtype evaluation of primary aldosteronism. The details are discussed in the text. APA, aldosterone-producing adenoma; AVS, adrenal venous sampling; CT, computed tomography; GRA, glucocorticoid-remediable aldosteronism; IHA, idiopathic hyperaldosteronism; PAH, primary adrenal hyperplasia. (Modified from Young and Hogan[6] by permission.)

Subtype Studies

The third management issue guides the therapeutic approach by distinguishing APA and PAH from IHA and GRA. Unilateral adrenalectomy in patients with APA or PAH results in normalization of hypokalemia in all and improved (nearly all) or cured (30% to 60%) hypertension.[43] In IHA and GRA, unilateral or bilateral adrenalectomy seldom corrects the hypertension.[40]

Primary aldosteronism subtype evaluation may require one or more tests, the first of which is imaging the adrenal with CT (FIG. 4). The mean diameter of the adenoma in 143 surgically treated APAs at our institution was 1.8 cm, although in nearly one-fifth (19%), it was <1 cm.[40] When a solitary unilateral macroadenoma (>1 cm) and normal contralateral adrenal morphology are found on CT in a young patient (<40 years) with primary aldosteronism, unilateral adrenalectomy is a reasonable therapeutic option (FIG. 4). However, in many cases, CT imaging may reveal normal-appearing adrenals, minimal unilateral adrenal limb thickening, unilateral microadenomas (≤1 cm), or bilateral macroadenomas. In these cases, additional testing is required to determine the source of excess aldosterone secretion. Small APAs may be labeled incorrectly as "IHA" on the basis of CT findings of bilateral nodularity or normal-appearing adrenals. Also, apparent adrenal microadenomas may represent areas of hyperplasia, and unilateral adrenalectomy would be inappropriate. In addition nonfunctioning unilateral adrenal macroadenomas are not uncommon, especially in older patients (>40 years of age).[44]

Patients with APAs have more severe hypertension, more profound hypokalemia (<3.0 mEq/L), higher plasma (>25 ng/dL) and urinary (>30 μg/24 hour) levels of aldosterone, and are of younger age (<50 years) than those with IHA.[40,45] Patients fitting these descriptors are considered to have a "high probability of APA" (FIG. 4). However, these factors are not absolute predictors of unilateral versus bilateral adrenal disease. With the addition of adrenal venous sampling, we have found unilateral APA in 36% of those with clinically "high-probability" APA who had normal findings or unilateral adrenal limb thickening on CT.[46] Gordon and colleagues reported that CT scanning contributed to lateralization in only 59 of 111 patients with surgically proven APA; CT picked up less than 25% of the APAs that measured less than 1 cm in diameter.[36] Magill and colleagues reported that in 38 patients who had both CT and adrenal venous sampling, CT imaging was either inaccurate or provided no additional information in 68% of their patients with primary aldosteronism.[47] Therefore, adrenal venous sampling is essential to direct appropriate therapy in patients with primary aldosteronism who have a high probability of APA and CT findings of unilateral adrenal limb thickening.

Adrenal Venous Sampling

Adrenal venous sampling is the gold standard test to differentiate unilateral from bilateral disease in the patient with primary aldosteronism.[48] Adrenal venous sampling is a difficult procedure because of the small right adrenal vein; the success rate is dependent on the proficiency of the angiographer.[36] The success rate at cannulating the right adrenal vein in 384 patients from 47 reports was 74%.[40] The success rate increases with experience to 90–93%.[36,46] At some centers adrenal venous sampling is performed in all patients diagnosed with primary aldosteronism.[36] A more practical approach is the selective use of adrenal venous sampling outlined in FIGURE 4. To minimize stress-induced fluctuations in aldosterone secretion, an infusion of 50 μg of cosyntropin per hour is initiated 30 minutes before adrenal vein catheterization and continued throughout the procedure.[46] The adrenal veins are catheterized via the percutaneous femoral venous approach, and the position of the catheter tip is verified by gentle injection of a small amount of nonionic contrast medium and radiographic documentation. Blood is obtained from both adrenal veins and the inferior vena cava (IVC) below the renal veins and assayed for aldosterone and cortisol concentrations. The venous sample from the left side typically is obtained from the inferior phrenic vein immediately adjacent to the entrance of the adrenal vein. Proper catheter placement should be confirmed by laboratory analyses of the blood samples showing high concentrations of cortisol in the adrenal vein as compared with that in the IVC.[46] The diagnostic criteria for determining a unilateral source of aldosterone are reported elsewhere.[46] Among patients with normal findings or minimal thickening of an adrenal limb on CT, 36% had a unilateral source of aldosterone discovered by adrenal venous sampling.[46] In patients with apparent unilateral microadenomas on CT, 50% had APAs.[46] In patients with bilateral adrenal abnormalities on CT, 37% had a unilateral source of aldosterone on adrenal venous sampling.[46]

Subtype Evaluation Tests of Historical Interest

Multiple tests and procedures were used to distinguish between APA and IHA before the development of the combined adrenal CT and adrenal venous sampling approach summarized above. At the Mayo Clinic, $[^{131}I]$-19-iodocholesterol scintigraphy was first used in 1973 and an improved agent, $[6\beta\text{-}^{131}I]$iodomethyl-19-norcholesterol (NP-59), was introduced in 1977.[49,50] The NP-59 scan, performed with dexamethasone suppression, had the advantage of correlating function with anatomical abnormalities. However, the sensitivity of this test depends heavily on the size of the adenoma.[51,52] Because tracer uptake is poor in adenomas < 1.5 cm in diameter, this method often is not helpful in interpreting micronodular findings obtained with high-resolution CT. The posture stimulation test, also developed in the 1970s, is based on the finding that blood aldosterone levels in patients with APA show a diurnal variation and are relatively unaffected by changes in angiotensin II levels.[53] In contrast, IHA is characterized by enhanced sensitivity to a small change in angiotensin II that occurs with standing. In a review of 16 reports in the literature, the accuracy of the posture stimulation test was 85% in 246 patients with surgically verified APA.[40] However, it became clear that some APAs are sensitive to angiotensin II and that some patients with IHA have diurnal variation in aldosterone secretion.[54] Also, although the posture stimulation test may predict which patient has APA, it does not assist in localization. Serum 18-hydroxycorticosterone (18-OHB) is considered to be either the immediate precursor of aldosterone or a separate end-product formed after 18-hydroxylation of corticosterone.[55] Patients with APA generally have recumbent serum 18-OHB levels greater than 100 ng/dL at 0800 hours, whereas in patients with IHA the levels are usually less than 50 ng/dL.[56–58] The diagnostic accuracy of 18-OHB for APA is approximately 82%.[40] Serum 18-OHB levels serve as a surrogate for plasma aldosterone that is also higher in patients with APA vs. IHA.

It has become clear that, beyond historical interest, there is no role for many of the tests that have been standards in the subtype evaluation of primary aldosteronism (e.g., NP-59 scintigraphy, posture stimulation test, and serum 18-OHB concentration).

FAMILIAL ALDOSTERONISM

Familial hyperaldosteronism type I is glucocorticoid-remediable and should be suspected in the following clinical situations: (1) primary aldosteronism is diagnosed in the first to third decades of life; (2) there is a family history of primary aldosteronism; or (3) there is a family history of cerebrovascular events at a young age (18% of 167 proven GRA patients have suffered cerebrovascular complications at an average age of 32 years).[59] The majority of these patients are normokalemic, a finding most likely explained by the diurnal nature of this disorder: "ACTH-dependent aldosterone excess by day and eualdosteronism by night."[60] A 24-hour urine 18-hydroxycortisol excretion in excess of 3000 nmol or direct genetic blood testing with Southern blotting or a long polymerase chain reaction technique to detect the chimeric gene confirm the diagnosis.[19,61,62]

Familial hyperaldosteronism type II is an autosomal dominant disorder of both IHA and APA. Thus far, 17 FH II families (with 44 affected members) have been reported. In at least seven families, dominant inheritance is suggested.[63] In a recent study, 7 patients from one kindred were screened for CYP11B1/CYP11B2 and CYP11B2 (aldo synthase gene on chromosome 8q), and all were negative for the defect.[63,64] A genome-wide search was recently completed in a large family with FH II, and genetic linkage was identified with the polymorphic markers D7S511, D7S517, and GATA24F02 on chromosome 7 (7p22).[65] The gene responsible for FH Type II has not yet been identified.

TREATMENT

The goal of treatment is to prevent morbidity and mortality associated with hypertension and hypokalemia. The cause of the primary aldosteronism determines the appropriate treatment. Although hypertension is frequently cured with unilateral adrenalectomy in patients with APA and PAH, the average cure rate for IHA is only 19% after unilateral or bilateral adrenalectomy.[40] IHA and GRA should be treated medically.

Surgical Treatment of APA and PAH

Although treatment of APAs with venous infarction and radiofrequency ablation have been reported,[66] the treatment of choice for APA and PAH is unilateral total adrenalectomy. The preoperative blood pressure response to spironolactone often predicts the blood pressure response to unilateral adrenalectomy in patients with APA. Indeed, APA patients who want to avoid surgery may be treated lifelong with an aldosterone receptor antagonist.[67] To decrease the surgical risk, hypokalemia should be corrected with an aldosterone receptor antagonist (e.g., spironolactone) before the operation. Laparoscopic adrenalectomy is the surgical approach of choice and is associated with shorter hospital stays and less long-term morbidity than occurs with the unilateral posterior or open abdominal approaches.[68] Unilateral adrenalectomy obviates the need for corticosteroid coverage.

Typically, the hypertension takes 1 to 6 months to resolve. Although nearly 100% of patients have improved blood pressure control postoperatively, average long-term cure rates with unilateral adrenalectomy for APA are 30% to 60%.[6,43] We analyzed the surgical treatment outcomes in 93 consecutive patients with primary aldosteronism treated with unilateral adrenalectomies at Mayo Clinic.[43] Hypertension was resolved at follow-up (blood pressure < 140/90 mm Hg) without use of antihypertensive agents in 31 of 93 patients (33%). According to a stepwise multivariable logistic regression analysis adjusted for duration of follow-up, resolution of hypertension was independently associated with family history of hypertension in no more than one first-degree relative (odds ratio [OR], 10.9; $P < 0.001$) and preoperative use of two or fewer antihypertensive agents (OR, 4.7; $P = 0.005$). Additional factors associated with resolution of hypertension based on univariate analysis included younger age, shorter duration of hypertension, higher preoperative ratio of plasma aldosterone concentration to plasma renin activity, and higher urine aldosterone level ($P < 0.05$).[43]

Pharmacological Treatment of IHA

Dietary sodium restriction (<100 mEq sodium/day), maintenance of ideal body weight, alcohol avoidance, and regular aerobic exercise contribute significantly to the success of pharmacologic treatment. Potassium supplementation in the form of medication or as a diet rich in potassium is usually ineffective in correcting the hypokalemia of primary aldosteronism. Although spironolactone often controls the hypertension and hypokalemia, it also blocks both testosterone biosynthesis and peripheral androgen action. Impotence, decreased libido, gynecomastia, menstrual irregularities, and minor gastrointestinal tract symptoms can all result. Amiloride (Midamor) is the drug of choice if patients are intolerant of spironolactone.

Eplerenone is a new specific aldosterone receptor antagonist that is in Phase III clinical trials. When compared to spironolactone, eplerenone has 0.1% of the binding affinity to androgen receptors.[69] The effectiveness of eplerenone in the treatment of mild to moderate essential hypertension has been demonstrated.[70] Eplerenone will be the superior drug if it is shown to be as effective as spironolactone for treatment of mineralocorticoid-dependent hypertension and if it lacks the limiting anti-androgen side effects of spironolactone.

If hypertension persists despite adequate tolerable doses of the potassium-sparing diuretic, a second-step agent should be added. Hypervolemia is a major reason for drug resistance in primary aldosteronism. Low doses of a thiazide or related sulfonamide diuretic add to blood pressure control when used in combination with the potassium-sparing diuretic. If a third agent is needed, a calcium channel blocker such as nifedipine is a reasonable choice. Nifedipine has also been shown to lower aldosterone secretion from APAs.[71]

REFERENCES

1. CONN, J.W. 1955. Presidential address: Part I. Painting background; Part II. Primary aldosteronism, a new clinical syndrome. J. Lab. Clin. Med. **45**: 3–17.
2. GORDON, R.D., M. STOWASSER, T.J. TUNNY, et al. 1994. High incidence of primary aldosteronism in 199 patients referred with hypertension. Clin. Exp. Pharmacol. Physiol. **21**: 315–318.
3. LOH, K., E. KOAY, M. KHAW, et al. 2000. Prevalence of primary aldosteronism among Asian hypertensive patients in Singapore. J. Clin. Endocrinol. Metab. **85**: 2854–2859.
4. YOUNG, W.F., JR. 1999. Primary aldosteronism: a common and curable form of hypertension. Cardiol. Rev. **7**: 207–214.
5. STOWASSER, M. 2001. Primary aldosteronism: rare bird or common cause of secondary hypertension? Curr. Hypertens. Rep. **3**: 230–239.
6. YOUNG, W.F., JR. & M.J. HOGAN. 1994. Renin-independent hypermineralocorticoidism. Trends Endocrinol. Metab. **5**: 97–106.
7. GANGULY, A. 1998. Primary aldosteronism. N. Engl. J. Med. **339**: 1828–1834.
8. IRONY, I., C.E. KATER, E.G. BIGLIERI, et al. 1990. Correctable subsets of primary aldosteronism: primary adrenal hyperplasia and renin responsive adenoma. Am. J. Hypertens. **3**: 576–582.
9. LIFTON, R.P., R.G. DLUHY, M. POWERS, et al. 1992. A chimaeric 11β-hydroxylase/aldosterone synthase gene causes glucocorticoid-remediable aldosteronism and human hypertension. Nature 355: 262–265.
10. DLUHY, R.G. 2001. Glucocorticoid-remediable aldosteronism. Endocrinologist **11**: 263–268.
11. TANABE, A., M. NARUSE, K. NARUSE, et al. 1997. Left ventricular hypertrophy is more prominent in patients with primary aldosteronism than in patients with other types of secondary hypertension. Hypertens. Res. **20**: 85–90.
12. ROSSI, G.P., A. SACCHETTO, E. PAVAN, et al. 1997. Remodeling of the left ventricle in primary aldosteronism due to Conn's adenoma. Circulation. **95**: 1471–1478.
13. SHIGEMATSU, Y., M. HAMADA, H. OKAYAMA, et al. 1997. Left ventricular hypertrophy precedes other target-organ damage in primary aldosteronism. Hypertension. **29**: 723–727.

14. HALIMI, J.M. & A. MIMRAN. 1995. Albuminuria in untreated patients with primary aldosteronism or essential hypertension. J. Hypertens. **13:** 1801–1802.
15. TORRES, V.E., W.F. YOUNG, JR., K.P. OFFORD, et al. 1990. Association of hypokalemia, aldosteronism, and renal cysts. N. Engl. J. Med. **322:** 345–351.
16. DUPREZ, D., M. DE BUYZERE, E.R. RIETZCHEL, et al. 2000. Aldosterone and vascular damage. Curr. Hypertens. Rep. **2:** 327–234.
17. NISHIMURA, M., T. UZU, T. FUJII, et al. 1999. Cardiovascular complications in patients with primary aldosteronism. Am. J. Kidney. Dis. **33:** 261–266.
18. STREETEN, D.H., N. TOMYCZ, & G.H. ANDERSON. 1979. Reliability of screening methods for the diagnosis of primary aldosteronism. Am. J. Med. **67:** 403–413.
19. RICH, G.M., S. ULICK, S. COOK, et al. 1992. Glucocorticoid-remediable aldosteronism in a large kindred: clinical spectrum and diagnosis using a characteristic biochemical phenotype. Ann. Intern. Med. **116:** 813–820.
20. GALLAY, B.J., S. AHMAD, L. XU, et al. 2001. Screening for primary aldosteronism without discontinuing hypertensive medications: plasma aldosterone-renin ratio. Am. J. Kidney. Dis. **37:** 699–705.
21. HIRAMATSU, K., T. YAMADA, Y. YUKIMURA, et al. 1981. A screening test to identify aldosterone-producing adenoma by measuring plasma renin activity: results in hypertensive patients. Arch. Intern. Med. **141:** 1589–1593.
22. MCKENNA, T.J., S.J. SEQUEIRA, A. HEFFERANAN, et al. 1991. Diagnosis under random conditions of all disorders of the renin-angiotensin-aldosterone axis, including primary hyperaldosteronism. J. Clin. Endocrinol. Metab. **73:** 952–957.
23. BROWN, M.A., H.A. CRAMP, V.C ZAMMIT, et al. 1996. Primary hyperaldosteronism: a missed diagnosis in "essential hypertensives"? Aust. N. Z. J. Med. **26:** 533–538.
24. FARDELLA, C., L. MOSSO, C. GOMEZ-SANCHEZ, et al. 2000. Primary hyperaldosteronism in essential hypertensives: prevalence, biochemical profile, and molecular biology. J. Clin. Endocrinol. Metab. **85:** 1863–1867.
25. GORDON, R.D., M.D. ZIESAK, T.J. TUNNY, et al. 1993. Evidence that primary aldosteronism may not be uncommon: 12% incidence among antihypertensive drug trial volunteers. Clin. Exp. Pharmacol. Physiol. **20:** 296–298.
26. HAMLET, S.M., T.J. TUNNY, E. WOODLAND, et al. 1985. Is aldosterone/renin ratio useful to screen a hypertensive population for primary aldosteronism? Clin. Exp. Pharmacol. Physiol. **12:** 249–252.
27. KREZE, A., D. OKALOVA, P. VANUGA, et al. 1999. [Occurrence of primary aldosteronism in a group of ambulatory hypertensive patients.] Vnitr. Lek. **45:** 17–21 [Slovak].
28. KUMAR, A., S.B. LALL, A. AMMINI, et al: 1994. Screening of a population of young hypertensives for primary hyperaldosteronism. J. Hum. Hypertens. **8:** 731–732.
29. LAZUROVA, I., P. SCHWARTZ, D. TREJBAL, et al. 1999. [Incidence of primary hyperaldosteronism in hospitalized hypertensive patients.] Bratisl. Lek. Listy. **100:** 200–203 [Slovak].
30. LIM, P., E. DOW, R. JUNG, et al. 2000. Prevalence of primary aldosteronism in the Tayside hypertension clinic population. J. Hum. Hypertens. **14:** 311–315.
31. LIM, P.O., P. RODGERS, K. CARDALE, et al. 1999. Potentially high prevalence of primary aldosteronism in a primary-care population. Lancet. **353:** 40.
32. MOSSO, L., C. FARDELLA, J. MONTERO, et al. 1999. [High prevalence of undiagnosed primary hyperaldosteronism among patients with essential hypertension.] Rev. Med. Chile. **127:** 800–806 [Spanish].

33. ROSSI, G.P., E. ROSSI, E. PAVAN, *et al.* 1998. Screening for primary aldosteronism with a logistic multivariate discriminant analysis. Clin. Endocrinol. **49:** 713–723.
34. MONTORI, V.M. & W.F. YOUNG, JR. 2002. Use of plasma aldosterone concentration-to-plasma renin Aactivity ratio as a screening test for primary aldosteronism. A systematic review of the literature. Endocrinol. Metab. Clin. N. Amer. In press.
35. MONEVA, M.H. & C.E. GOMEZ-SANCHEZ. 2001. Establishing a diagnosis of primary aldosteronism. Curr. Opin. Endocrinol. Diab. **8:** 124–129.
36. GORDON, R.D., M. STOWASSER & J.C. RUTHERFORD. 2001. Primary aldosteronism: are we diagnosing and operating too few patients? World J. Surg. **25:** 941–947.
37. MONTORI, V.M., G.L. SCHWARTZ, A.B CHAPMAN, *et al.* 2001. Validity of the aldosterone-renin ratio used to screen for primary aldosteronism. Mayo Clin. Proc. **76:** 877–882.
38. HIROHARA, D., K. NOMURA, T. OKAMOTO, *et al.* 2001. Performance of the basal aldosterone to renin ratio and of the renin stimulation test by furosemide and upright posture in screening for aldosterone-producing adenoma in low renin hypertensives. J. Clin. Endocrinol. Metab. **86:** 4292–4298.
39. WEINBERGER, M.H. & N.S. FINEBERG. 1993. The diagnosis of primary aldosteronism and separation of two major subtypes. Arch. Int. Med. **153:** 2125–2129.
40. YOUNG, W.F., JR & G.G KLEE. 1988. Primary aldosteronism: diagnostic evaluation. Endocrinol. Metab. Clin. N. Amer. **17:** 367–395.
41. HOLLAND, O., H. BROWN, L. KUHNERT, *et al.* 1984. Further evaluation of saline infucion for the diagnosis of primary aldosteronism. Hypertension **6:** 717–723.
42. BRAVO, E.L., R.C. TARAZI, H.P. DUSTAN, *et al.* 1983. The changing clinical spectrum of primary aldosteronism. Am. J. Med. **74:** 641–651.
43. SAWKA, A.M., W.F. YOUNG, JR., G.B. THOMPSON, *et al.* 2001. Primary aldosteronism: factors associated with normalization of blood pressure after surgery. Ann. Intern. Med. **135:** 258–261.
44. KLOOS, R.T., M.D. GROSS, I.R. FRANCIS, *et al:* 1995. Incidentally discovered adrenal masses. Endocr. Rev. **16:** 460–484.
45. BLUMENFELD, J.D., J.E. SEALEY, Y. SCHLUSSEL, *et al.* 1994. Diagnosis and treatment of primary aldosteronism. Ann. Intern. Med. **121:** 877–885.
46. YOUNG, W.F. JR, A.W. STANSON, C.S. GRANT, *et al.* 1996. Primary aldosteronism: adrenal venous sampling. Surgery **120:** 913–920.
47. MAGILL, S.B., H. RAFF, J.L. SHAKER, *et al.* 2001. Comparison of adrenal vein sampling and computed tomography in the differentiation of primary aldosteronism. J. Clin. Endocrino.l Metab. **86:** 1066–1071.
48. MAGILL, S.B. 2001. Adrenal vein sampling: an overview. Endocrinologist **11:** 357–363.
49. CONN, J.W., W.H. BEIERWALTES, L.M. LIEBERMAN, *et al.* 1971. Primary aldosteronism: preoperative tumor visualization by scintillation scanning. J. Clin. Endocrinol. Metab. **33:** 713–716.
50. MILES, J.M., H.W. WAHNER, P.C. CARPENTER, *et al.* 1979. Adrenal scintiscanning with NP-59, a new radioiodinated cholesterol agent. Mayo. Clin. Proc. **54:** 321–327.

51. HOGAN, M.J., J. MCRAE, M. SCHAMBELAN, et al. 1976. Location of aldosterone-producing adenomas with 131I-19-iodocholesterol. N. Engl. J. Med. **294:** 410–414.
52. NOMURA, K., K. KUSAKABE, M. MAKI, et al. 1990. Iodomethylnorcholesterol uptake in an aldosteronoma shown by dexamethasone-suppression scintigraphy: relationship to adenoma size and functional activity. J. Clin. Endcrinol. Metab. **71:** 825–830.
53. GANGULY, A., A.J. DOWDY, J.A. LUETSCHER, et al. 1973. Anomalous postural response of plasma aldosterone concentration in patient with aldosterone-producing adrenal adenoma. J. Clin. Endocrinol. Metab. **36:** 401–404.
54. IRONY, I., C.E. KATER, E.G. BIGLIERI, et al. 1990. Correctable subsets of primary aldosteronism. Primary adrenal hyperplasia and renin responsive adenoma. Am. J. Hypertens. **3:** 576–382.
55. FRASER, R. & C.P. LANTOS. 1978. 18-Hydroxycorticosterone: a review. J. Steroid Biochem. **9:** 273–286.
56. BIGLIERI, E.G. & M. SCHAMBELAN. 1979. The significance of elevated levels of plasma 18-hydroxycorticosterone in patients with primary aldosteronism. J. Clin. Endocrinol. Metab. **49:** 87–91.
57. KEM, D.C., K. TANG, C.S. HANSON, et al. 1985. The prediction of anatomical morphology of primary aldosteronism using serum 18-hydroxycorticosterone levels. J. Clin. Endocrinol. Metab. **60:** 67–73.
58. PHILLIPS, J.L., M.M. WALTHER, J.C. PEZZULLO, et al. 2000. Predictive value of preoperative tests in discriminating bilateral adrenal hyperplasia from an aldosterone-producing adenoma. J. Clin. Endocrinol. Metab. **85:** 4526–4533.
59. LITCHFIELD, W.R., B.F. ANDERSON, R.J. WEISS, et al. 1998. Intracranial aneurysm and hemorrhagic stroke in glucocorticoid-remediable aldosteronism. Hypertension. **31:** 445–450.
60. LITCHFIELD, W.R., C. COOLIDGE, P. SILVA, et al. 1997. Impaired potassium-stimulated aldosterone production: a possible explanation for normokalemic glucocorticoid-remediable aldosteronism. J. Clin. Endocrinol. Metab. **82:** 1507–1510.
61. MULATERO, P., F. VEGLIO, C. PILON, et al. 1998. Diagnosis of glucocorticoid-remediable aldosteronism in primary aldosteronism: aldosterone response to dexamethasone and long polymerase chain reaction for chimeric gene. J. Clin. Endocrinol. Metab. **83:** 2573–2575.
62. STOWASSER, M., M.G. GARTSIDE, & R.D. GORDON. 1997. A PCR-based method of screening individuals of all ages, from neonates to the elderly, for familial hyperaldosteronism type I. Aust. N. Z. J. Med. **27:** 685–690.
63. GORDON, R.D., D.J. TORPY, A.R. LAFFERTY, et al. 1999. Familial hyperaldosteronism type II (FH-II) [abstract #S55-2]. *In* Program and Abstracts of 81st Annual Meeting of the Endocrine Society. San Diego. :54.
64. TORPY, D.J., R.D. GORDON, J.P. LIN, et al. 1998. Familial hyperaldosteronism type II: description of a large kindred and exclusion of the aldosterone synthase (CYP11B2) gene. J. Clin. Endocrinol. Metab. **83:** 3214–3218.
65. LAFFERTY, A.R., D.J. TORPY, M. STOWASSER, et al. 2000. A novel genetic locus for low renin hypertension: familial hyperaldosteronism type II maps to chromosome 7 (7p22). J. Med. Genet. **37:** 831–835.
66. KIGURE, T., T. HARADA, Y. SATOH, et al. 1996. Microwave ablation of the adrenal gland: experimental study and clinical application. Br. J. Urol. **77:** 215–220.

67. LIM, P.O., W.F. YOUNG, & T.M. MACDONALD. 2001. A review of the medical treatment of primary aldosteronism. J. Hypertens. **19:** 353–361.
68. THOMPSON, G.B., C.S. GRANT, J.A. VAN HEERDEN, *et al.* 1997. Laparoscopic versus open posterior adrenalectomy: a case-control study of 100 patients. Surgery. **122:** 1132–1136.
69. DE GASPARO, M., U. JOSS, H.P. RAMJOUE, *et al.* 1987. Three new epoxyspironolactone derivatives: characterization in vivo and in vitro. J. Pharmacol. Exp. Ther. **240:** 650–656.
70. EPSTEIN, M., J. MENARD, J.C. ALEXANDER, *et al.* 1998. Eplerenone, a novel and selective aldosterone receptor antagonist: efficacy in patients with mild to moderate hypertension. Circulation. **98**(Suppl)**:** I-98–99 [abstract 498].
71. YOKOYAMA, T., K. SHIMAMOTO, & O. IIMURA. 1995. Mechanism of inhibition of aldosterone secretion by Ca2+ channel blocker in patients with essential hypertension and patients with primary aldosteronism. Nippon Naibunpi Gakkai Zasshi **71:** 1059–1074.

New Genetic Insights in Familial Hyperaldosteronism

RICHARD V. JACKSON, ANTHONY LAFFERTY, DAVID J. TORPY, AND CONSTANTINE STRATAKIS

University of Queensland, Department of Medicine, Greenslopes Hospital, Brisbane, Queensland 4120, Australia

ABSTRACT: Aldosterone, the major circulating mineralocorticoid, particiates in blood volume and serum potassium homeostasis. Primary aldosteronism is a disorder characterized by hypertension and, in more severe form, hypokalemia, due to autonomous aldosterone secretion from the adrenocortical zona glomerulosa. Improved screening techniques, particularly application of the plasma aldosterone: plasma renin activity ratio, has led to renewed interest in Conn's original proposal that primary aldosteronism may be the cause of increased blood pressure in about 10% of adults with hypertension. Glucocorticoid-remediable aldosteronism (GRA) was the first described familial form of hyperaldosteronism. The disorder is characterized by aldosterone secretory function regulated chronically by ACTH. Hence, aldosterone hypersecretion can be chronically suppressed by exogenous glucocorticoids such as dexamethasone in physiologic-range doses. This autosomal dominant disorder has been shown to be caused by a hybrid gene mutation formed by a cross-over of genetic material between the ACTH-responsive regulatory portion of the 11β-hydroxylase (CYP11B1) gene and the coding region of the aldosterone synthase (CYP11B2) gene. Familial hyperaldosteronism type II (FH-II), so named to distinguish the disorder from GRA or familial hyperaldosteronism type I (FH-I), is characterized by inheritance consistent with an autosomal dominant pattern of autonomous aldosterone hypersecretion which is not suppressible by dexamethasone. Linkage analysis in a single large kindred, and direct mutation screening, has shown that this disorder is unrelated to mutations in the genes for aldosterone synthase or the angiotensin II receptor. A recent genome-wide search has identified a genetic linkage between FH-II in this single large kindred and polymorphic gene markers on chromosome 7 in a region that corresponds to cytogenetic band 7p22. This is the first identified locus for FH-II. Several possible candidate genes have been localized to the 7p22 region. The precise genetic cause of FH-II remains to be elucidated.

Address for correspondence: Rick Jackson, Associate Professor, Department of Medicine, University of Queensland, Greenslopes Private Hospital, Newdegate Street, Brisbane, Qld, 4120 Australia.

r.jackson@mailbox.uq.edu.au

KEYWORDS: primary aldosteronism; familial; genetics; diagnosis; glucocorticoid-remediable hyperaldosteronism; FH-II

INTRODUCTION

Aldosterone, the major circulating mineralocorticoid, is a steroid hormone produced exclusively in the zona glomerulosa in a series of six biosynthetic steps. The product of the CYP11B2 gene is capable of catalyzing the 11β-hydroxylase, 18-hydroxylase, and 18-hydroxydehydrogenase steps in aldosterone biosynthesis.[1,2] The CYP11B2 gene is located on human chromosome 8q24.3-tel, in close proximity to the highly homologous CYP11B1 gene, which codes only for the 11β-hydroxylase enzyme, and catalyzes the final step in cortisol synthesis.[3] At the level of the zona glomerulosa, the major stimulatory influences are angiotensin II and serum potassium concentration.[4,5] Adrenocorticotropic hormone (ACTH) stimulates aldosterone secretion in an acute and transient fashion, but ACTH probably does not play a direct role in the chronic regulation of aldosterone secretion.[6,7] The major inhibitory influences affecting the zona glomerulosa are exerted by circulating atrial natriuretic peptide (ANP)[8] and, locally, by dopamine.[9] Aldosterone acts on its target tissues (distal renal tubule, sweat glands, salivary glands, large intestinal epithelium) via its own specific mineralocorticoid receptors.[10,11] Mineralocorticoid receptors exhibit equal affinity for aldosterone and glucocorticoids,[12] but distal renal tubular receptors are protected from the effects of cortisol by 11β-hydroxysteroid dehydrogenase, which converts cortisol to inactive cortisone. A number of aldosterone precursors, including deoxycorticosterone and 18-hydroxycorticosterone, have mineralocorticoid activity, and their hypersecretion in various pathologic states may produce or exacerbate features typical of mineralocorticoid hypertension.

Hyperaldosteronism is characterized by excessive secretion of aldosterone with consequent increased sodium reabsorption and potassium and hydrogen ion excretion. Clinical features include hypertension, hypokalemia, and metabolic alkalosis. Cardiovascular fibrosis has been related to aldosterone hypersecretion.[13–15]

Hyperaldosteronism represents a subset of disorders known as mineralocorticoid hypertension. These include two rare causes of congenital adrenal hyperplasia (11β-hydroxylase deficiency and 17α-hydroxylase deficiency), the syndrome of apparent mineralocorticoid excess (AME) due to 11β-hydroxysteroid dehydrogenase (11β-HSD) deficiency, primary glucocorticoid resistance, Liddle's syndrome, and exogenous sources of mineralocorticoid such as licorice or drugs such as carbenoxolone. The features of mineralocorticoid excess are also often seen in Cushing's syndrome, particularly in patients with ectopic ACTH-producing tumors. In these cases, it is postulated that excessive glucocorticoid levels overwhelm the ability of the 11β-HSD enzyme to inactivate cortisol at the kidney mineralocorticoid receptor level.

PRIMARY ALDOSTERONISM

Primary aldosteronism was originally described by J.W. Conn[16] as a syndrome of hypertension associated with hypokalemia and postulated hypersecretion of an endogenous mineralocorticoid. Early reported cases were due to an aldosterone-producing adrenocortical adenoma (APA), removal of which led to some of the earliest cures of hypertension.[17]

Earlier reliance on plasma potassium as a screening test, as advocated by some authorities,[18] may have led to under-recognition of the contribution of primary aldosteronism to hypertension. An early study, using saline infusion as a screening test for primary aldosteronism, reported a frequency of 2.2% of primary aldosteronism among 1,036 unselected hypertensives,[19] but recent studies using the ratio of plasma aldosterone to plasma renin activity (ARR) concentrations in plasma suggested that primary aldosteronism may account for at least 8.5% of hypertensives.[20–25] The use of laparoscopic adrenalectomy has reduced the morbidity of surgery for APA.[26] Primary aldosteronism is most frequently diagnosed in middle-aged adults, is more common in women, and is rare in children.

DIAGNOSIS OF PRIMARY ALDOSTERONISM

The currently advocated diagnostic process follows the sequence of screening, confirmation of aldosterone secretory autonomy, differential diagnosis (unilateral surgically remediable or bilateral source of aldosterone), and exclusion of FH-I.[27] The validity of screening for primary aldosteronism with the plasma aldosterone: renin activity ratio (ARR), performed under random conditions with respect to salt intake, is now well-documented.[28–30] There is not universal agreement about the validity of the ARR's being used to screen for primary aldosteronism because the ARR does not provide a renin-independent measure of circulating aldosterone.[31,32] There is no consensus regarding the indications for screening among hypertensives which takes into account recent reports of increased prevalence of primary aldosteronism using the ARR. The presence of hypertension and hypokalemia predicts primary aldosteronism with 50% accuracy,[31] but normokalemic hypertensive primary aldosteronism is now well recognized. Factors that may lead to misleading ARR tests need to be taken into account, including diuretics, spironolactone, β-blockers, dihydropyridine calcium channel blockers, renal impairment and untreated hypokalaemia. Several tests have been advocated for confirmation of aldosterone secretory autonomy including the intravenous saline suppression test,[19] the oral salt/fludrocortisone suppression test,[21] the oral salt-loading test with measures of 24-hr urine aldosterone excretion,[34] or the oral captopril test.[35,36] These tests have not been rigorously compared.[37] In some cases with very high ARR tests, confirmation of aldosterone secretory capacity may not be necessary.

Differential diagnosis, primarily between bilateral adrenal hyperplasia (BAH) and aldosterone-producing adenoma (APA), can be achieved with postural testing, where BAH exhibits a rise in aldosterone with upright posture indicative of responsiveness to angiotensin II.[38] 18-hydroxycorticosterone levels,[38,39] adrenal computed tomograms (70% sensitivity for APA, coexistent incidentalomas may confound this test), and adrenal venous sampling, which remains the gold standard test despite some controversy over technique and interpretation.[40–44] Uncommon forms of primary aldosteronism include angiotensin-II-responsive APA, which shows an aldosterone response to posture or angiotensin II infusion, glucocorticoid-remediable aldosteronism, which can be excluded with specific genetic testing or a dexamethasone suppression test, and primary adrenal hyperplasia, where unilateral autonomous aldosterone secretion occurs without a discrete tumor on gland resection.[41,45]

Familial forms of hyperaldosteronism include familial hyperaldosteronism type I (glucocorticoid-remediable aldosteronism) and familial hyperaldosteronism type II. Hyperaldosteronism has also been seen in multiple endocrine neoplasia type-1 (MEN-I).[46]

FAMILIAL HYPERALDOSTERONISM TYPE I

In 1966, the first familial cases of hypertension due to a dexamethasone-suppressible form of hyperaldosteronism were reported.[47] This autosomal dominant disease is known as glucocorticoid-remediable aldosteronism (GRA) or, recently, familial hyperaldosteronism type I (FH-I). GRA is characterized by bilateral adrenal hyperplasia, or rarely, adrenal adenoma.[48] GRA accounts for approximately 1% of cases of primary hyperaldosteronism.

The genetic locus for this disorder was recently established by genetic linkage analysis and the causative mutation subsequently identified.[49] The defect involves a crossover of genetic material between the closely related highly homologous genes that code for the enzyme 11β-hydroxylase (CYP11B1) (which catalyzes the last step in cortisol biosynthesis) and the gene for aldosterone synthesis (CYP11B2). Fusion of a portion of the regulatory region of CYP11B1, the ACTH-responsive promoter, with the coding region of the CYP11B2 gene, allows aldosterone synthesis to be strongly directed by ACTH, resulting in pathologically high levels of aldosterone and extreme suppressibility of aldosterone to exogenous glucocorticoid administration.

Elucidation of this mutation readily explained the cardinal pathophysiological features of the disorder. The synthesis of "hybrid" steroids, 18-oxocortisol and 18-hydroxycorticosterone, requires the action of 17α-hydroxylase on aldosterone, an enzyme expressed only in the zona fasciculata, suggesting that aldosterone is synthesized in the zona fasciculata in this disorder.[50] Higher blood pressure in the offspring of affected mothers rather than affected fathers has been attributed to the effects of high maternal aldosterone on the fetus rather than imprinting.[51,52] Importantly, not all individuals with the GRA mutation have hypertension, and ongoing studies of the physiologic and genetic bases of their counterbalancing hypotensive systems are in progress.[53] The lack of hypokalemia in many subjects with GRA has been related to a blunted aldosterone response to potassium, which may reduce the severity of hyperaldosteronism.[54] Availability of a genetic test for GRA has allowed exploration of the phenotype, such as demonstration of the association of intracranial aneurysm and haemorrhagic stroke with GRA.[55]

FAMILIAL HYPERALDOSTERONISM TYPE II

Familial hyperaldosteronism type II as a distinct entity was recognized by R.D. Gordon,[21,56] although other isolated familial cases of non-dexamethasone-suppressible hyperaldosteronism have also been reported.[57,58] In addition, we are aware of several other families with non-dexamethasone-suppressible familial hyperaldosteronism, from a variety of other countries. After initial serendipitous discovery of two cases in a single family, subsequent cases have been identified by application of the ARR screening test followed by confirmatory testing, and surgery if indicated. To date, 17 families (44 individuals) with FH-II have been identified by the Gordon group.[59] All families are of Caucasian descent, from a variety of European backgrounds. There has been no clinical or biochemical evidence of multiple endocrine neoplasia type I in the affected families. Families with APA alone, BAH, or both entities represented in one family have been detected. The age range at diagnosis was 14–72 years.

The FH-II phenotype is clinically indistinguishable from a large control group of cases of sporadic primary aldosteronism assembled by Gordon *et al.* with respect to age of onset, gender, frequency of hypokalemia, aldosterone, and PRA levels, and relative frequency of APA and IHA.[59] In contrast to FH-I, where genetic testing is available, and autosomal dominant inheritance is well established, the mode of inheritance of FH-II remains speculative. However, in the large kindred reported elsewhere, vertical transmission suggests autosomal dominant inheritance. This is also the case in six other FH-II families. In the largest FH-II kindred reported, X-linked inheritance cannot be excluded on segregation analysis, although linkage analysis involving microsatellites on the X-chromosome has been negative.

Our genetic studies of FH-II have focussed on a single large kindred with seven family members who suffer from hyperaldosteronism. Hyperaldosteronism has been demonstrated by the use of the ARR in all cases and by fludrocortisone suppression testing in six of the seven affected individuals. The five hypertensive subjects with primary aldosteronism had adrenal venous sampling results indicative of bilateral adrenal autonomous aldosterone production. Hence, adrenalectomy was not justified and tumor tissue was not available from this family. For genetic linkage analysis purposes, those with positive ARR tests and nonsuppression of aldosterone levels on fludrocortisone suppression testing were classified as affected, hypertensive individuals with normal ARR or those younger than 20 were classified a "query" affected, and normotensive individuals with normal ARR and age greater than 20 were classified as unaffected.[56]

A number of candidate genes were studied, based on physiologically based hypotheses regarding the possible etiology of FH-II. These hypotheses included the possibility of activating mutations of the angiotensin II type I receptor gene and the CYP11B2 "aldosterone synthase" gene. We excluded involvement of the angiotensin II type 1 receptor gene in FH-II by means of genetic linkage analysis using a dinucleotide (CA) repeat polymorphism contained in a 0.9Kb Eco RI fragment approximately 15Kb downsteam from the 5′ end of the AT1 gene coding sequence.[60]

Although the hybrid gene mutation which causes FH-I had tested negative by PCR[61] and/or Southern blot technique in all cases, an activating mutation of CYP11B2, different from the hybrid gene mutation seen in FH-I, could cause FH-II.[62] Accurate chromosomal localization of the CYP11B2 gene was achieved by radiation hybrid mapping and fluorescent *in situ* hybridization.[3] We then excluded involvement of the CYP11B2 gene in the FH-II phenotype of the single large kindred using a poly-A repeat marker within the 5′ region of the CYP11B2 gene and nine other markers in an 80cM region extending from 8q21-8qtel.[56] The LOD score for the CYP11B2 intragenic marker was −12.6 at a recombination distance (θ) of 0.

A number of other candidate genes were excluded from segregation with the FH-II phenotype in this family, including the MEN1 locus at chromosome 11q13. Although loss of heterozygosity (LOH) at the 11q13 chromosomal locus has been described in APA, including those from FH-II patients, LOH at this locus is a frequent finding in sporadic endocrine tumours. Recently, a genome-wide search was completed.[63] Most of the genome was excluded. A locus was identified on the short arm of chromosome 7 corresponding to the cytogenetic band 7p22 (FIG.1) to which our large kindred maps with a peak

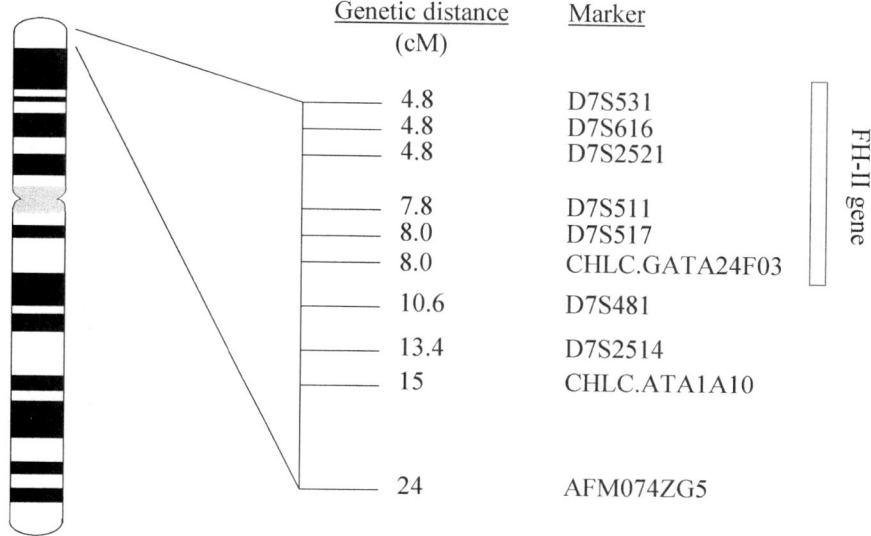

FIGURE 1.

two-point lod score of 3.26 at a recombination fraction of zero. Multipond linkage analysis yielded a peak lod score of 3.5. This area of chromosome 7 is telomeric in location and is not well represented in existing genome maps. Hence, the only available polymorphic markers from 7p22 are the ones used in this study. Candidate genes are either involved in tumorigenesis or have a possible role in central or peripheral regulation of the renin–angiotensin system. These candidate genes are: (1) GPR30, a G-protein–coupled receptor; (2) PMS2, the human homologue of a S.cerevisiae postmeiotic segregation gene; (3) PRKAR1B, a cyclic AMP–dependent protein kinase regulatory protein type 1β; and (4) Centaurin-alpha 1 gene.

PRKAR1B is the favored candidate gene. It forms a heterotetramer when it binds with the catalytic subunits of protein kinase A (PKA). PRKAR1A is the gene coding for the regulatory subunit type 1A of PKA and is a functional partner of type 1B. Type 1A is mutated in the Carney complex, which is associated with adrenocortical tumors producing glucocorticoids.[64] No candidate genes with a functional link to aldosterone synthase were identified.

FH-II is the fourth genetically determined cause of hypermineralocorticoidism to be identified. The other three causes are GRA (FH-I), 11β-hydroxylase deficiency (where DOC is increased) and 17α-hydroxylase deficiency (also characterized by an increase in DOC). Elucidation of the causative gene in FH-II may have implications for both sporadic primary aldosteronism and hypertension in general, as well as providing insight into the regulation of blood pressure in general.

CONCLUSIONS

Familial primary aldosteronism has offered opportunities to understand the genetic mechanisms underlying at least a subset of primary aldosteronism. This may be of importance in sporadic primary aldosteronism, which is being recognized with increasing frequency due to the application of plasma ARR testing in normokalemic hypertensives. The advent of laparoscopic adrenalectomy has reduced the morbidity of surgical treatment of primary aldosteronism. The unremarkable clinical features of FH-II so far ascertained relative to sporadic primary aldosteronism suggest that biochemical screening of family members of patients with primary aldosteronism should be employed more widely. With increasing recognition, a need to optimize diagnostic strategies will become evident. The place of screening for PAL among hypertensives has not yet received critical cost–benefit analysis. The gene for familial hyperaldosteronism type II has been localized to the short arm of chromosome 7 at position 7p22.

REFERENCES

1. MORNET, E., J. DUPONT, A. VITEK, et al. 1989. Characterisation of the two genes encoding human steroid 11β-hydroxylase (P-450 (11)β). J. Biol. Chem. **264:** 20961–20967.
2. CURNOW, K.M., M.T. TUSIE-LUNA, L. PASCOE, et al. 1991. The product of the CYP11B2 gene is required for aldosterone biosynthesis in the human adrenal cortex. Mol. Endocrinol. **5:** 1513–1522.
3. TAYMANS, S.E., S. PACK, E. PAK, et al. 1998. Human CYP11B2 (aldosterone synthase) maps to chromosome 8q24.3. J. Clin. Endocrinol. Metab. **83:** 1033–1036.
4. MCKENNA, T.J., D.P. ISLAND, W.E. NICHOLSON, et al. 1978. The effect of potassium on early and late steps in aldosterone biosynthesis in cells of the zona glomerulosa. Endocrinology **103:** 141.
5. CLYNE, C.D., Y. ZHANG, L. SLUTSKER, et al. 1997. Angiotensin II and potassium regulate human CYP11B2 transcription through common cis-elements. Mol. Endocrinol. **11:** 638–649.
6. BROWN, J.J., D.L. DAVIES & A.F. LEVER. 1964. Variations in plasma renin concentration in several physiological and pathological states. Can. Med. Assoc. J. **90:** 201.
7. GAILLARD, R.C., A.M. RIONDEL, C.A. FARROD-COUNE, et al. 1983. Aldosterone escape to chronic ACTH administration in man. Acta Endocrinol. (Copenh.) **103:** 116.
8. BLAIR-WEST, J.R., J.P. COUGHLIN & D.A. DENTON. 1980. A dose response comparison of the actions of angiotensin II and III in sheep. J. Endocrinol. **87:** 409.

9. CAREY, R.M. 1982. Acute dopaminergic inhibition of aldosterone secretion is independent of angiotensin II and adrenococrticotropin. J. Clin. Endocrinol. Metab. **54:** 463–469.
10. SHEPPARD, K.E. & J.W. FUNDER. 1987. Equivalent affinity of aldosterone and corticosterone for type I receptors in kidney and hippocampus: direct binding studies. J. Steroid Biochem. **28:** 737.
11. SHEPPARD, K.E. & J.W. FUNDER. 1987. Type I receptors in parotid, colon, and pituitary and aldosterone selective in vivo. Am. J. Physiol. **253:** E467.
12. FUNDER, J.W. 1995. Apparent mineralocorticoid excess. Endocrinol. Metab. Clin. N. Amer. **24:** 613-621.
13. CAMPBELL, S.E., A.A. DIAZ-ARIAS & K.T. WEBER. 1992. Fibrosis of the human heart and systemic organs in adrenal adenoma. Blood Pres. **1:** 149–156.
14. SUN, Y., F.J. RAMIRES & K.T. WEBER. 1997. Fibrosis of atria and great vessels in response to angiotensin II or aldosterone infusion. Cardiovasc. Res. **35:** 138–147.
15. ROBERT, V., C. HEYMES & J.S. SILVESTRE. 1999. Angiotensin AT1 receptor subtype as a cardiac target of aldosterone: role in aldosterone-salt-induced fibrosis. Hypertension **33:** 981–986.
16. CONN, J.W. 1995. Primary aldosteronism, a new clinical syndrome. J. Lab. Clin. Med. **45:** 3–17.
17. CONN, J.W., R.F. KNOPF & R.M. NESBIT. 1964. Clinical characteristics of primary aldosteronism from an analysis of 145 cases. Am. J. Surg. **107:** 159–172.
18. KAPLAN, N.M. 1992. Endocrine hypertension. *In* Williams Textbook of Endocrinology, 8th ed. :707–731. W.B. Saunders. Philadelphia.
19. STREETEN, D.H.P., N. TOMYCZ & G.H. ANDERSON, JR. 1979. Reliability of screening methods for the diagnosis of primary aldosteronism. Am. J. Med. **67:** 403–413.
20. GORDON, R.D., M. STOWASSER, T.J. TUNNY, *et al.* 1994. High incidence of primary hyperaldosteronism in 199 patients referred with hypertension. Clin. Exp. Pharmacol. Physiol. **21:** 315–418.
21. GORDON, R.D. 1995. Primary aldosteronism. J. Endocrinol. Invest. 18: 495–511.
22. FARDELLA, C.E., L. MOSSO, C.E. GOMEZ-SANCHEZ, *et al.* 2000. Primary hyperaldosteronism in essential hypertensives: prevalence, biochemical profile and molecular biology. J. Clin. Endocrinol. Metab. **85:** 1863–1867.
23. LIM, P.W., E. DOW, G. BRENNAN, *et al.* 2000. High prevalence of primary aldosteronism in the Tayside Hypertension Clinic population. J. Hum. Hypertens. **14:** 311–315.
24. LOH, K.C., E.S. KOAY, M.C. KHAW, *et al.* 2000. Prevalence of primary aldosteronism among Asian hypertensive patients in Singapore. J. Clin. Endocrinol. Metab. **85:** 2854–2859.
25. NISHIKAWA, T. & M. OMURA. 2000. Clinical characteristics of primary aldosteronism: its prevalence and comparative studies on various causes of primary aldosteronism in Yokohama Rosai Hospital. Biomed. Pharmacother. **54(Suppl 1):** 83s–85s.
26. WEISNAGEL, S.J., M. GAGNER, G. BRETON, *et al.* 1996. Laparoscopic adrenalectomy. The Endocrinologist **6:** 169–178.

27. LITCHFIELD, W.R. & R.G. DLUHY. 1995. Primary aldosteronism. Endocrinol. Metab. Clin. N. Amer. **24:** 593–612.
28. HIRAMATSU, K., T. YAMADA, Y. YUKIMURA, *et al.* 1981. A screeening test to identify aldosterone-producing adenoma by measuring plasma renin activity: results in hypertensive patients. Arch. Intern. Med. **141:** 1589–1593.
29. MCKENNA, T.J., S.J. SEQUEIRA, A. HEFFERNAN, et al. 1991. Diagnosis under random conditions of all disorders of the renin-angiotensin-aldosterone axis, including primary hyperaldosteronism. J. Clin. Endocrinol. Metab. 73: 952–957.
30. IGNATOWSKA-SWITALSKA, H., J. CHODAKOWSKA, W. JANUSZEWICZ, *et al.* 1997. Evaluation of plasma aldosterone to plasma renin activity ratio in patients with primary aldosteronism. J. Hum. Hypertens. **11:** 373–378.
31. MONTORI, V.M., G.L. SCHWARTZ, A.B. CHAPMAN, *et al.* 2001. Validity of the aldosterone-renin ratio used to screen for primary aldosteronism. Mayo Clin. Proc. **76:** 877–882.
32. KAPLAN, N.M. 2001. Caution about the overdiagnosis of primary aldosteronism. Mayo Clin. Proc. **76:** 875–876.
33. MELBY, J.C. 1991. Diagnosis of hyperalodsteronism. Endocrinol. Metab. Clin. N. Amer. **20:** 247–255.
34. BRAVO, E.L., R.C. TURAZI & H.P. DUSTAN. 1983. The changing clinical spectrum of primary aldosteronism. Am. J. Med. **74:** 641–651.
35. HAMBLING, C., R.T. JUNG, A. GUNN, *et al.* 1992. Re-evaluation of the captopril test for the diagnosis of primary hyperaldosteronism. Clin. Endocrinol. (Oxf.) **36:** 499–503.
36. IWAOKA, T., T. UMEDA, S. NAOMI, *et al.* 1993. The usefulness of the captopril test as a simultaneous screening for primary aldosteronism and renovascular hypertension. Am. J. Hypertens. **6:** 899–906.
37. GANGULY, A. 2001. Prevalence of primary aldosteronism in unselected hypertensive populations: screening and definitive diagnosis. J. Clin. Endocrinol. Metab. **86:** 4002–4003.
38. YOUNG, W.F., JR. & G.G. KLEE. 1988. Primary aldosteronism: diagnostic evaluation. Endocrinol. Metab. Clin. N. Amer. **17:** 367–395.
39. ULICK, S., J.D. BLUMENFIELD, S.A. ATLAS, *et al.* 1993. The unique steroidogenesis of the aldosteronoma in the differential diagnosis of primary aldosteronism. J. Clin. Endocrinol. Metab. **76:** 873-878.
40. DOPPMAN, J.L. & J.R. GILL, JR. 1996. Hyperaldosteronism: sampling the adrenal veins. Radiology **198:** 309–312.
41. YOUNG, W.F., JR. 1997. Primary hyperaldosteronism: update on diagnosis and treatment. The Endocrinologist **7:** 213–221.
42. PHILLIPS, J.L., M.M. WALTHER, J.C. PEZZULLO, *et al.* 2000. Predictive value of preoperative tests in discriminating bilateral adrenal hyperplasia from an aldosterone-producing adrenal adenoma. J. Clin. Endocrinol. Metab. **85:** 4526–4533.
43. MAGILL, S.B., H. RAFF, J.L. SHAKER, *et al.* 2001. Comparison of adrenal vein sampling and computed tomography in the differentiation of primary aldosteronism. J. Clin. Endocrinol. Metab. **86:** 1066–1071.
44. ROSSI, G.P., A. SACCHETTO, M. CHIESURA-CORONA, *et al.* 2001. Identification of the etiology of primary aldosteronism with adrenal vein sampling in patients with equivocal computed tomography and magnetic resonance

findings: results in 104 consecutive cases. J. Clin. Endocrinol. Metab. **86:** 1083–1090.
45. BIGLIERI, E.G. 1997. Primary aldosteronism. Curr. Ther. Endocrinol. Metab. **6:** 170–172.
46. BECKERS, A., R. ABS & P.J. WILLEMS. 1992. Aldosterone secreting adenoma as part of multiple endocrine neoplasia type 1 (MEN I): loss of heterozygosity for polymorphic chromosome 11 deoxyribonucleic acid markers, including the MEN I locus. J. Clin. Endocrinol. Metab. **75:** 564–570.
47. SUTHERLAND, D.J.A., J.C. RUSE & J.C. LAIDLAW. 1966. Hypertension increased aldosterone secretion and low plasma renin activity relieved by dexamethasone. J. Can. Med. Assoc. **95:**1109–1119.
48. PASCOE, L., X. JEUNEMAITRE, M.C. LEBRETHON, et al. 1995. Glucocorticoid-suppressible hyperaldosteronism and adrenal tumors occurring in a single French pedigree. J. Clin. Invest. **96:** 2236-2246.
49. LIFTON, R.P., R.G. DLUHY, M. POWERS, et al. 1992. A chimaeric 11β-hydroxylase/aldosterone synthase gene causes glucocorticoid-remediable aldosteronism and human hypertension. Nature **355:** 262–265.
50. ULICK, S. & M.D. CHU. 1982. Hypersecretion of a new corticosteroid, 18-hydroxycortisol in two types of adrenocortical hypertension. Clin. Exp. Hypertens. **A4:** 1771-1777.
51. JAMIESON, A., L. SLUTSKER, G.C. INGLIS, et al. 1995. Glucocorticoid suppressible hyperaldosteronism: effects of cross-over site and parental origin of chimaeric gene on phenotypic expression. Clin. Sci. **88:** 563–570.
52. WHITE, P.C. 1997. Abnormalities of aldosterone synthesis and action in children. Curr. Opin. Pediatr. **9:** 424–430.
53. GATES, L.J., A.A. MACCONNACHIE, R.P. LIFTON, et al. 1996. Variation of phenotype in patients with GRA. J. Med. Genet. **33:** 25–28.
54. LITCHFIELD, W.R,. M.I. NEW, C. COOLIDGE, et al. 1997. Evaluation of the dexamethasone suppression test for the diagnosis of glucocorticoid-remediable aldosteronism. J. Clin. Endocrinol. Metab. **82:** 3570–3573.
55. LITCHFIELD, W.R., B.F. ANDERSON, R.J. WEISS, et al. 1998. Intracranial aneurysm and hemorrhagic stroke in glucocorticoid-remediable aldosteronism. Hypertension **31:** 445–450.
56. TORPY, D.J., R.D. GORDON, J.-P. LIN, et al. 1998. Familial hyperaldosteronism type-II: description of a large kindred and exclusion of the aldosterone synthase (CYP11B2) gene. J. Clin. Endocrinol. Metab. **83:** 3214–3218.
57. LONDON, N., J. SWALES, K. HOLLINRAKE, et al. 1992. Familial Conn's syndrome. Postgrad. Med. J. **68:** 976–977.
58. GRECO, R.G., J.E. CARROLL, D.J. MORRIS, et al. 1982. Familial hyperaldosteronism, not suppressed by dexamethasone. J. Clin. Endocrinol. Metab. **55:** 1013–1016.
59. GORDON, R.D. & M. STOWASSER. 1998. Familial forms broaden the horizons for primary aldosteronism. Trends Endocrinol. Metab. **9:** 220–227.
60. TORPY, D.J., R.D. GORDON & C.A. STRATAKIS. 1998. Linkage analysis of familial hyperaldosteronism type II: absence of linkage to the gene encoding the angiotensin II receptor type 1. J. Clin. Endocrinol. Metab. **83:**1046.
61. JONSSON, J.R., S.A. KLEMM, T.J. TUNNY, et al. 1995. A new genetic test for familial hyperaldosteronism type 1 aids in the detection of curable hypertension. Biochem. Biophys. Res. Commun. **207:** 565–571.

62. KATOH, T., T. ISE, H. TAKAKUWA, *et al.* A new variant of familial hyperaldosteronism [abstract P1813]. Proceedings of the 14th International Congress on Nephrology, 1997.
63. LAFFERTY, A.R., D.J. TORPY, M. STOWASSER, *et al.* 2000. A novel genetic locus for low renin hypertension: familial hyperaldosteronism type II maps to chromosome 7 (7p22). J. Med. Genet. **37:** 831–835.
64. KIRSCHNER, L.S., J.A. CARNEY, S. PACK, *et al.* 2000. Mutations of the PRKAR1A gene in patients with Carney complex. Nat. Genet. **26:** 89–92.

The Pathophysiology of Aldosterone in the Cardiovascular System

RICARDO ROCHA[a] AND JOHN W. FUNDER[b]

[a]*Global Medical Affairs, Pharmacia Corporation, Peapack, New Jersey, USA*
[b]*Baker Medical Research Institute, Melbourne, Victoria, Australia*

ABSTRACT: Until relatively recently, the mineralocorticoid hormone aldosterone was thought to be produced uniquely in the adrenal cortex and to act exclusively on epithelia to promote sodium retention and potassium excretion. However, it is now known that aldosterone also acts on nonepithelial tissues, such as brain, heart, and blood vessels, and that enzymes required for aldosterone biosynthesis are expressed in these same tissues, which may be consistent with local aldosterone production acting in a paracrine fashion. A number of studies indicate that aldosterone exerts clearly deleterious effects when levels are inappropriate for salt status. For example, aldosterone in a high-salt environment initiates a vascular inflammation response that leads to cardiac and vascular pathologies. In experimental models of hypertension and heart failure, the nonepithelial effects of aldosterone are mediated via classical mineralocorticoid receptors, and are largely or completely abolished by administration of the selective aldosterone blocker eplerenone or by reduction of circulating aldosterone by adrenalectomy. In the present manuscript, we review some of the most recent discoveries in the field of aldosterone biology, with special emphasis on the mechanisms involved in the deleterious actions of this mineralocorticoid in cardiovascular tissues.

KEYWORDS: aldosterone; angiotensin II; eplerenone; hypertension; mineralocorticoids

INTRODUCTION

After decades of research on the mineralocorticoid aldosterone, a simple view developed in which the hormone was thought to act exclusively in the regulation of salt and volume homeostasis. According to this "classical" model, aldosterone is produced uniquely from the adrenal glomerulosa in re-

---

Address for correspondence: Ricardo Rocha, M.D., Associate Medical Director, Global Medical Affairs, Pharmacia Corporation, 100 Route 206 North, P.O. Box 800, Peapack, NJ. Voice: 908-901-8961; fax: 908-901-1945; mobile: 847-778-2744.
rrroch@pharmacia.com

sponse to angiotensin II, adrenocorticotropin hormone (ACTH), and potassium, and interacts with epithelial cells located in the distal nephron of the kidney, colon, and salivary and sweat glands. In the nephron, where the effects have been studied most thoroughly, aldosterone has been found to diffuse directly across the plasma membrane and to bind to the inactive cytoplasmic form of the mineralocorticoid receptor (MR). This binding dissociates the MR from a multiprotein complex containing molecular chaperones,[1] which in turn mediates translocation of the MR through the nuclear pores to the chromatin.[2] In the nucleus, the activated receptor acts as a positive transcription factor to modulate expression of multiple proteins, including the serum and glucocorticoid inducible kinase 1 (sgk-1).[3] Aldosterone-induced sgk-1 expression triggers a cascade of events that ultimately increases the absorption of Na^+ ions and water through the epithelial sodium channel and indirectly increases K^+ excretion.[4] Ultimately, at the end of this cascade, intravascular volume expands and blood pressure rises.

The preceding view of aldosterone remains substantially intact today, but a recent and ongoing revolution in our understanding of aldosterone biology has led to a deeper appreciation of "non-classical" aspects of the hormone.[5] For example, it is now clear that MRs are present not only in epithelial cells of the kidney, colon, and salivary and sweat glands, but also in epithelial and nonepithelial tissues like the heart,[6] brain,[7] and blood vessels.[8] Moreover, extra-adrenal synthesis of aldosterone in these same tissues has been documented, and a localized paracrine role has been proposed.[8–10] It is also now clear that aldosterone secretion can be elevated by mechanisms independent of angiotensin II, a previously suspected degree of redundancy.[11–15] Finally, aldosterone levels that are inappropriate for salt status (elevated or within the normal range) are now known to result in marked pathophysiologic sequelae mediated by MR in both epithelial and nonepithelial tissues. All of these results suggest that the "classical" view of aldosterone, that is, a hormone involved exclusively in salt/volume homeostasis, needs considerable expansion.

The last ten years also witnessed an expanded appreciation of aldosterone in the clinic. The glucocorticoid-remediable aldosteronism (GRA) syndrome was elucidated at the molecular level in 1992.[16] This syndrome is characterized by an unusually high incidence of cerebrovascular accidents, often lacking associated hypokalemia.[17,18] For many years, primary aldosteronism (PAL) was believed to be a rare form of secondary hypertension. However, this disease has been shown to occur at a higher incidence than previously thought.[19–27] Broader use of diagnostic tools like the plasma aldosterone/renin ratio, followed by bilateral renal venous catheterization, indicates that 5%–20% of unselected "essential" hypertensive patients have PAL. Many of these patients (particularly those presenting with bilateral adrenal adenomas) are normokalemic, as is the case in patients with GRA, and some even have aldosterone levels within what is considered to be the normal range. It is interesting that these patients have been shown to have a significant incidence of left ventricular hypertrophy,[28] microalbuminuria,[29] and stroke,[30] arguing against the common belief that this is a rather benign form of secondary hypertension.

The most compelling evidence indicating the harmful effects of aldosterone on the cardiovascular system comes from the Randomized Aldactone Evaluation Study (RALES) reported in 1999.[31] This randomized, double-blind study showed that the addition of a low dose of the nonselective aldosterone blocker, spironolactone, to current best-practice treatment of patients with severe heart failure (NYHA Class III-IV) improved mortality and morbidity by a remarkable 30% and 35%, respectively. This, again, argues for a major role of aldosterone in the pathophysiology of cardiovascular disease that requires a much better understanding.

CARDIOVASCULAR PROTECTION AND ALDOSTERONE BLOCKADE: EFFECTS ON THE HEART

A number of studies have demonstrated that the heart may be a potential site of extra-adrenal aldosterone production. Highly sensitive molecular approaches have identified aldosterone biosynthetic enzymes and aldosterone itself in cardiac tissues, although considerable variation has been observed across and within species and under different pathophysiologic circumstances.[10,32,33] In one study, myocardial infarction raised aldosterone synthase mRNA by 2.0-fold and aldosterone levels by 3.7-fold in non-infarcted myocardium, and these increases were completely blocked by angiotensin II type I receptor (AT-1) inhibitors, suggesting that this receptor is responsible for activating cardiac aldosterone synthesis.[34] Given the extreme sensitivity required for these assays, however, it is perhaps not surprising that other studies have reached different conclusions. For example, two studies in humans concluded it was unlikely that aldosterone played a significant autocrine or paracrine role in the heart.[35,36] Moreover, in humans, conflicting reports of aldosterone production in the failing heart have yet to be reconciled.[33,36]

Regardless of how the preceding conundrum is eventually resolved, accumulating evidence has documented the deleterious effects of systemic aldosterone in the heart.

Pioneering studies from Karl Weber's laboratory have shown that systemic infusion of aldosterone at 0.75 μg/hr to uninephrectomized rats drinking 0.9% NaCl solution raised blood pressure and caused cardiac hypertrophy with both right and left ventricular fibrosis[37,38] (FIG. 1). Neither hypertension nor the cardiac effects were seen in rats on a low-salt diet. Importantly, a low dose of MR antagonist reversed the cardiac effects of the administered aldosterone with minimal changes in blood pressure.

A similar blood pressure-independent and protective effect of aldosterone antagonism in the heart has been observed in other hypertensive animal models, such as the L-NAME/Ang II hypertensive rat, which does not display hyperaldosteronemia.[39] In this model, either administration of eplerenone, a selective aldosterone blocker (SAB), or adrenalectomy significantly reduced coronary vascular injury without lowering blood pressure. Notably, the protective effect of adrenalectomy was completely abolished by aldosterone replacement via subcutaneous infusion. Therefore, adrenal gland mineralocorticoids play a major role in the development of vascular injury in the hypertensive rat heart. A similar effect of aldosterone antagonism was recently reported in the double transgenic renin/angiotensinogen rat.[40] These data demonstrate that aldosterone, in the presence of a high-salt environment, has the ability to induce coronary vascular damage through mechanisms independent of blood pressure.

A fact that remains puzzling is the intensifying role of a high-salt/volume environment for the deleterious effects of aldosterone in the cardiovascular system. It was in the early 1940s that Friedman[41] and, separately, Selye,[42] reported that addition of a high-salt diet or renal mass reduction augmented and accelerated (without qualitatively altering) the pathologic effects of mineralocorticoids in cardiovascular tissues. The mechanisms for this relationship between salt and aldosterone remain unclear. However, this relationship becomes clinically relevant when patients display plasma aldosterone levels that are inappropriate for the amount of dietary salt consumption or the magnitude of intravascular volume. Indeed, patients presenting any degree of volume retention or those consuming a high-salt diet should demonstrate very low levels of circulating aldosterone. This ability to inhibit aldosterone synthesis can be abnormally reduced, as in the case of patients with heart failure who commonly present secondary aldosteronism, despite concurrent intravascular volume overload.

The mechanisms by which aldosterone contributes to the development of cardiovascular injury are the focus of recent investigations. A recent animal study has looked into the effects of aldosterone at the level of the coronary vasculature.[43] Uninephrectomized rats receiving a high-salt diet and aldosterone developed severe hypertension after two weeks of treatment. Histological examination demonstrated marked vascular inflammatory lesions, characterized by fibrinoid necrosis of the media and associated perivascular inflammatory cell infiltration. The lesions were evident after as few as two weeks of aldosterone treatment and became more frequent and severe with time. The infiltrating cells were primarily macrophages, as suggested by positive staining with an ED-1 monoclonal antibody. Immunohistochemistry and/or *in situ* hybridization identified an augmented expression of VCAM-1

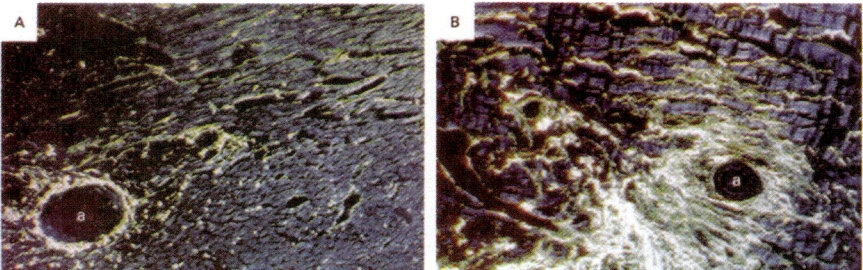

FIGURE 1. Myocardium from (**A**) normal rat and from (**B**) a rat receiving chronic aldosterone/salt treatment showing significant perivascular and interstitial fibrosis. a: artery. (From Weber.[50] Reproduced with permission.)

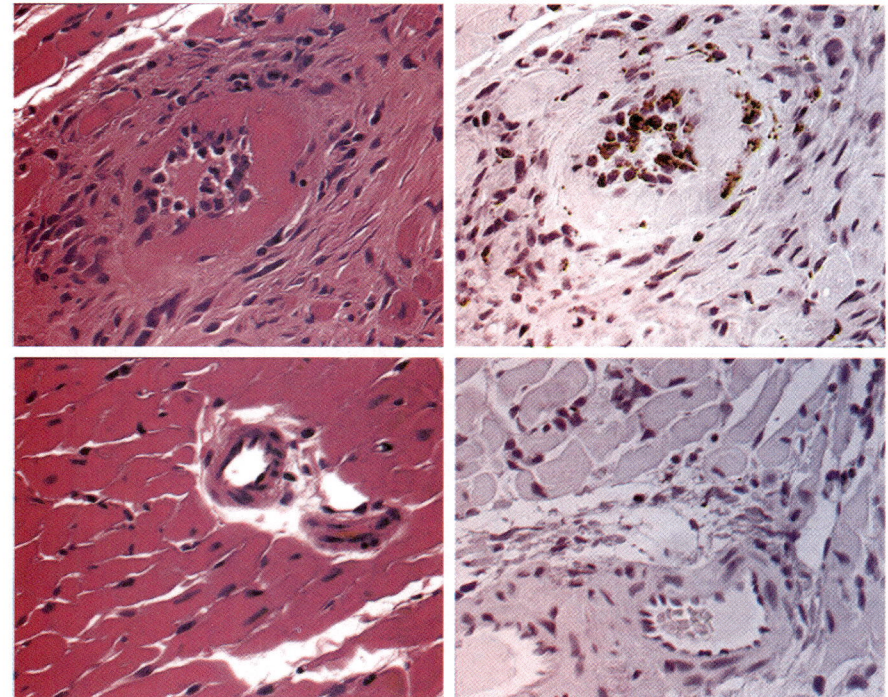

FIGURE 2. *Upper left:* Representative coronary lesion induced by aldosterone/salt treatment showing fibrinoid necrosis of the media accompanied by a severe perivascular inflammatory response (hematoxylin and eosin stain; original magnification 400×). *Upper right:* Same lesion as at left immunostained with the macrophage-specific monoclonal antibody, ED-1. The majority of cells infiltrating the lesions were identified as macrophages. *Lower left:* Myocardium of an animal receiving aldosterone/salt treatment in the presence of the selective aldosterone blocker, eplerenone, showing no lesions. *Lower right:* Myocardium of an eplerenone-treated rat immunostained with the macrophage-specific monoclonal antibody, ED-1.

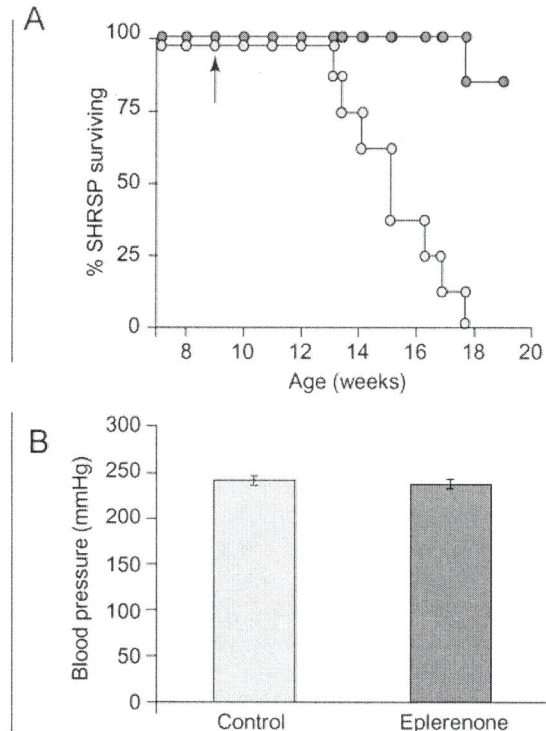

FIGURE 3. (**A**) Survival curves for SHRP treated with vehicle (light circles, $n = 8$) or eplerenone (dark circles, $n = 7$; 100 mg kg^{-1}; $P < 0.001$). *Arrow* indicates when treatment began. (**B**) Systolic blood pressure in SHRSP receiving either vehicle (*light bar*) or eplerenone (*dark bar*) (P + n.s.). (From Rocha and Steier.[5] Reproduced by permission.)

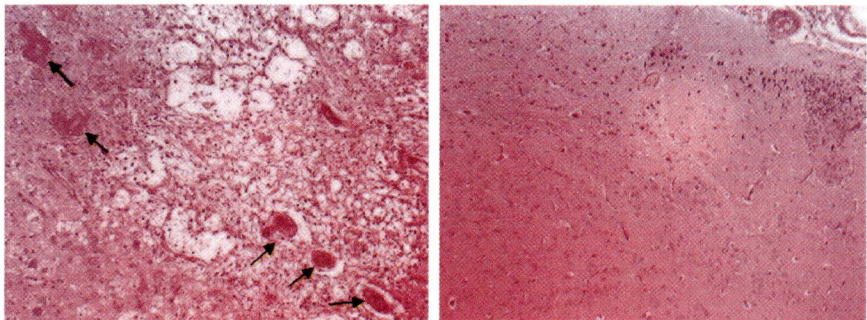

FIGURE 4. Cerebral histopathology with or without eplerenone. *Left:* Photomicrograph of cerebral cortex of a stroke-prone, spontaneously hypertensive rat (SHRSP) receiving vehicle treatment, showing fibrinoid necrotic lesions in cerebral arteries (*arrows*) and liquefaction necrosis in the parenchyma. *Right:* Cerebral cortex of a SHRSP receiving eplerenone treatment and showing no damage. Scale bars = 80 μm.

in the coronary endothelium, and an augmented expression of COX-2 and the chemokine osteopontin in the media. Consistently, mRNA expression for COX-2, osteopontin, and MCP-1, another chemokine, was elevated after one week of treatment, and levels progressively increased with time.

Administration of eplerenone resulted in a significant reduction in blood pressure, vascular damage, and associated inflammatory changes. Consistently, eplerenone substantially reduced the tissue expression of inflammatory molecules in the heart. A representative photomicrograph of the coronary inflammatory lesions induced by aldosterone is shown in FIGURE 2.

The previous results demonstrate that vascular inflammation and associated damage/necrosis arise early in uninephrectomized rats treated with high salt and aldosterone. Selective aldosterone blockade with eplerenone can dramatically attenuate these effects. These data are consistent with the hypothesis that aldosterone receptor stimulation produces vascular inflammation, which subsequently leads to myocardial ischemia, necrosis, and fibrosis.

Eplerenone similarly attenuated the progressive decline in myocardial function and LV chamber remodeling in dogs with established heart failure induced with multiple coronary microembolizations.[44] Three months of therapy with this selective aldosterone blocker induced a substantial fall in left ventricular end-diastolic pressure, maintained left ventricular end-diastolic volume, and markedly reduced left ventricular end-diastolic wall stress. Myocyte size and interstitial collagen levels were significantly higher in untreated dogs, and capillary density was correspondingly lower, which is further evidence for the protective effects of eplerenone in the abnormal remodeling process that characterizes the progression of heart failure in this model. More importantly, the progressive decline in left ventricular ejection fraction observed in untreated controls was prevented by three months of therapy with eplerenone.

Thus, in a variety of settings, selective aldosterone blockade appears to confer beneficial cardiovascular effects, not only by reducing the levels of hypertension, but also by preventing the structural remodeling that occurs in the heart and coronary vasculature. These observations are in agreement with the RALES trial, which previously underscored the potential benefit of aldosterone antagonism in patients with heart failure.

CARDIOVASCULAR PROTECTION AND ALDOSTERONE BLOCKADE: EFFECTS ON THE BRAIN

As described previously, various areas of the brain, most notably the hypothalamus, appear capable of aldosterone biosynthesis.[9] The significance of this has yet to be fully elucidated, but several recent studies indicate that MRs in the brain are biologically and clinically relevant. In particular, a direct role for aldosterone in the regulation of blood pressure in the brain has been identified. Indeed, local intracerebroventricular (i.c.v.) infusions of aldosterone at a dose of 10 ng/hr, a dose without physiological effects when infused peripherally, elevated blood pressure in saline-drinking, uninephrectomized rats to levels at least as high as those seen with a systemic infusion of aldosterone at 1 µg/hr.[45] Consistently, the severe elevation in blood pressure observed during aldosterone/salt hypertension was prevented by local i.c.v. infusions of the MR antagonist RU28318, even at doses too low to reduce blood pressure when administered systemically. Another recent study has also identified a potential role for aldosterone in the central regulation of salt appetite.[46]

Another potentially deleterious effect of aldosterone in the central nervous system has been identified in the stroke-prone, spontaneously hypertensive rat (SHRSP). These rats, derived from the original Okamoto-SHRs, develop a malignant hypertension syndrome within 7–10 weeks of initiation of a high-salt, potassium-deficient diet. The syndrome is characterized by stroke and severe nephrosclerosis and is accompanied by a paradoxical activation of the renin–angiotensin–aldosterone system (RAAS), despite the presence of a high-salt diet. The rats die primarily from stroke between 13 and 18 weeks of age.

SHRSP treated from 9 weeks of age with the SAB eplerenone were protected against the development of stroke and malignant nephrosclerosis and survived for a significantly longer period of time compared with vehicle-treated littermates (7 of 8 alive at 19 weeks [FIG. 3A]).[47] The protective effect was seen despite the fact that eplerenone-treated animals remained as hypertensive as the vehicle-treated controls (FIG. 3B). Histopathological examination of the brains in the eplerenone-treated SHRSP showed marked attenuation of cerebral injury (FIG. 4). Thus, aldosterone appears to play a major role in the development of cerebrovascular disease in hypertensive rats, independent of its effects on blood pressure. The mechanisms underlying this role remain to be elucidated, but may be related to the ability of aldosterone to induce abnormal remodeling of the vasculature, as we have previously shown in the heart.

CARDIOVASCULAR PROTECTION AND ALDOSTERONE BLOCKADE: EFFECTS IN THE KIDNEY

As described above, malignant nephrosclerosis correlates with the elevated renin and aldosterone levels that characterize SHRSP.[47] Administration of eplerenone or spironolactone[48] to SHRSP markedly reduced urinary protein excretion and renal vascular lesions. While kidney sections from vehicle-treated SHRSP showed glomerulosclerosis, dilated tubules, abundant casts, and fibrinoid necrosis of the medium- and small-sized renal arteries, renal damage was significantly reduced by aldosterone blockade, despite the presence of severe hypertension. A similar protective effect on the kidney has been previously demonstrated with ACE inhibition in this model. However, the protection of ACE inhibition can be effectively reduced by administration of exogenous infusions of aldosterone.[49] This suggests a pivotal role for aldosterone in the pathophysiology of nephrosclerosis that may be independent of angiotensin II or other components of the RAAS. If true, it further underscores the potential therapeutic benefits of selective aldosterone blockade for treatment of hypertensive renal disease.

SUMMARY

Aldosterone, which now appears to be synthesized not only in adrenal glomerulosa but also at other extra-adrenal sites, interacts with epithelial and nonepithelial tissues outside of the kidney, colon, and sweat and salivary glands. Some of these interactions clearly play a role in the regulation of blood pressure and salt and volume homeostasis, both at the level of the CNS as well as in epithelial tissues. Others, however, can be maladaptive and can lead to significant vascular lesions in target organs. Aldosterone in a high-salt environment, for example, induces a vascular inflammatory response characterized by perivascular leukocyte infiltration, vascular remodeling with fibrinoid necrosis of the media, and consequent ischemic and necrotic alterations in the tissues compromised. This response could be the first step in the development of cardiac fibrosis, hypertensive nephrosclerosis, or stroke. The nonepithelial effects of systemic or locally produced aldosterone are largely or completely abolished by administration of selective aldosterone blockers. Thus, accumulating evidence indicates that aldosterone, in the presence of a high-salt environment, plays a significant role in the pathophysiologic changes that occur in target organs of hypertensive disease.

REFERENCES

1. TRAPP, T. & F. HOLSBOER. 1995. Ligand-induced conformational changes in the mineralocorticoid receptor analyzed by protease mapping. Biochem. Biophys. Res. Commun. **215:** 286–291.
2. FEJES-TOTH, G., D. PEARCE & A. NARAY-FEJES-TOTH. 1998. Subcellular localization of mineralocorticoid receptors in living cells: effects of receptor agonists and antagonists. Proc. Natl. Acad. Sci. USA. **95:** 2973–2978.
3. CHEN, S.Y., A. BHARGAVA, L. MASTROBERARDINO, et al. 1999. Epithelial sodium channel regulated by aldosterone-induced protein sgk. Proc. Natl. Acad. Sci. USA. **96:** 2514–2519.
4. BHARGAVA, A., M.J. FULLERTON, K. MYLES, et al. 2001. The serum- and glucocorticoid-induced kinase is a physiological mediator of aldosterone action. Endocrinology **142:** 1587–1594.

5. ROCHA, R. & C.T. STIER, JR. 2001. Pathophysiological effects of aldosterone in cardiovascular tissues. Trends Endocrinol. Metab. **12:** 308–314.
6. LOMBES, M., N. ALFAIDY, E. EUGENE, et al. 1995. Prerequisite for cardiac aldosterone action. Mineralocorticoid receptor and 11 beta-hydroxysteroid dehydrogenase in the human heart. Circulation **92:** 175–182.
7. ROLAND, B.L., Z.S. KROZOWSKI & J.W. FUNDER. 1995. Glucocorticoid receptor, mineralocorticoid receptors, 11 beta- hydroxysteroid dehydrogenase-1 and -2 expression in rat brain and kidney: in situ studies. Mol. Cell Endocrinol. **111:** R1–7.
8. TAKEDA, Y., I. MIYAMORI, S. INABA, et al. 1997. Vascular aldosterone in genetically hypertensive rats. Hypertension **29(1 Pt 1):** 45–48.
9. GOMEZ-SANCHEZ, C.E., M.Y. ZHOU, E.N. COZZA, et al. 1997. Aldosterone biosynthesis in the rat brain. Endocrinology **138:** 3369–3373.
10. SILVESTRE, J.S., V. ROBERT, C. HEYMES, et al. 1998. Myocardial production of aldosterone and corticosterone in the rat. Physiological regulation. J. Biol. Chem. **273:** 4883–4891.
11. SATO, A. & T. SARUTA. 2001. Aldosterone escape during angiotensin-converting enzyme inhibitor therapy in essential hypertensive patients with left ventricular hypertrophy. J. Int. Med. Res. **29:** 13–21.
12. STRUTHERS, A.D. 1996. Aldosterone escape during angiotensin-converting enzyme inhibitor therapy in chronic heart failure. J. Card. Fail. **2:** 47–54.
13. PITT, B. 1995. "Escape" of aldosterone production in patients with left ventricular dysfunction treated with an angiotensin converting enzyme inhibitor: implications for therapy. Cardiovasc. Drugs Ther. **9:** 145–149.
14. BORGHI, C., S. BOSCHI, E. AMBROSIONI, et al. 1993. Evidence of a partial escape of renin-angiotensin-aldosterone blockade in patients with acute myocardial infarction treated with ACE inhibitors. J. Clin. Pharmacol. **33:** 40–45.
15. HALL, J.E., J.P. GRANGER, M.J. SMITH, JR. & A.J. PREMEN. 1984. Role of renal hemodynamics and arterial pressure in aldosterone "escape." Hypertension **6(2 Pt 2):** I183–192.
16. LIFTON, R.P., R.G. DLUHY, M. POWERS, et al. 1992. A chimaeric 11 beta-hydroxylase/aldosterone synthase gene causes glucocorticoid-remediable aldosteronism and human hypertension. Nature **355:** 262–265.
17. LITCHFIELD, W.R., R.G. DLUHY, R.P. LIFTON & G.M. RICH. 1995. Glucocorticoid-remediable aldosteronism. Compr. Ther. **21:** 553–558.
18. RICH, G.M., S. ULICK, S. COOK, et al. 1992. Glucocorticoid-remediable aldosteronism in a large kindred: clinical spectrum and diagnosis using a characteristic biochemical phenotype. Ann. Intern. Med. **116:** 813–820.
19. RAYNER, B.L., J.E. MYERS, L.H. OPIE, et al. 2001. Screening for primary aldosteronism--normal ranges for aldosterone and renin in three South African population groups. S. Afr. Med. J. **91:** 594–599.
20. GANGULY, A. 2001. Prevalence of primary aldosteronism in unselected hypertensive populations: screening and definitive diagnosis. J. Clin. Endocrinol. Metab. **86:** 4002–4004.
21. RAYNER, B.L., L.H. OPIE & J.S. DAVIDSON. 2000. The aldosterone/renin ratio as a screening test for primary aldosteronism. S. Afr. Med. J. **90:** 394–400.
22. LOH, K.C., E.S. KOAY, M.C. KHAW, et al. 2000. Prevalence of primary aldosteronism among Asian hypertensive patients in Singapore. J. Clin. Endocrinol. Metab. **85:** 2854–2859.

23. NISHIKAWA, T. & M. OMURA. 2000. Clinical characteristics of primary aldosteronism: its prevalence and comparative studies on various causes of primary aldosteronism in Yokohama Rosai Hospital. Biomed. Pharmacother. **54** (Suppl. 1): 83s–85s.
24. FARDELLA, C.E., L. MOSSO, C. GOMEZ-SANCHEZ, et al. 2000. Primary hyperaldosteronism in essential hypertensives: prevalence, biochemical profile, and molecular biology. J. Clin. Endocrinol. Metab. **85**: 1863–1867.
25. LIM, P.O., E. DOW, G. BRENNAN, et al. 2000. High prevalence of primary aldosteronism in the Tayside Hypertension Clinic population. J. Hum. Hypertens. **14**: 311–315.
26. LIM, P. O., P. RODGERS, K. CARDALE, et al. 1999. Potentially high prevalence of primary aldosteronism in a primary-care population. Lancet. **353**: 40.
27. ABDELHAMID, S., H. MULLER-LOBECK, S. PAHL, et al. 1996. Prevalence of adrenal and extra-adrenal Conn syndrome in hypertensive patients. Arch. Intern. Med. **156**: 1190–1195.
28. ROSSI, G.P., A. SACCHETTO, P. VISENTIN, et al. 1996. Changes in left ventricular anatomy and function in hypertension and primary aldosteronism. Hypertension. **27**: 1039–1045.
29. HALIMI, J.M. & A. MIMRAN. 1995. Albuminuria in untreated patients with primary aldosteronism or essential hypertension. J. Hypertens. **13(12 Pt 2)**: 1801–1802.
30. TAKEDA, R., T. MATSUBARA, I. MIYAMORI, et al. 1995. Vascular complications in patients with aldosterone producing adenoma in Japan: comparative study with essential hypertension. The Research Committee of Disorders of Adrenal Hormones in Japan. Jpn. Endocrinol. Invest.. **18**: 370–373.
31. PITT B., F. ZANNAD, W. J. REMME, et al. 1999. The effect of spironolactone on morbidity and mortality in patients with severe heart failure. Randomized Aldactone Evaluation Study Investigators. N. Engl. J. Med. **341**: 709–717.
32. TAKEDA, Y., T. YONEDA, M. DEMURA, et al. 2000. Cardiac aldosterone production in genetically hypertensive rats. Hypertension. **36**: 495–500.
33. MIZUNO, Y., M. YOSHIMURA, H. YASUE, et al. 2001. Aldosterone production is activated in failing ventricle in humans. Circulation **103**: 72–77.
34. SILVESTRE, J.S., C. HEYMES, A. OUBENAISSA, et al. 1999. Activation of cardiac aldosterone production in rat myocardial infarction: effect of angiotensin II receptor blockade and role in cardiac fibrosis. Circulation **99**: 2694–2701.
35. KAYES-WANDOVER, K.M. & P. C. WHITE. 2000. Steroidogenic enzyme gene expression in the human heart. J. Clin. Endocrinol. Metab. **85**: 2519–2525.
36. YOUNG, M.J., C.D. CLYNE, T.J. COLE & J.W. FUNDER. 2001. Cardiac steroidogenesis in the normal and failing heart. J. Clin. Endocrinol. Metab. **86**: 5121–5126.
37. BRILLA, C.G. & K.T. WEBER. 1992. Reactive and reparative myocardial fibrosis in arterial hypertension in the rat. Cardiovasc. Res. **26**: 671–677.
38. BRILLA, C.G., R. PICK, L.B. TAN, et al. 1990. Remodeling of the rat right and left ventricles in experimental hypertension. Circ. Res. **67**: 1355–1364.
39. ROCHA, R., C.T. STIER, JR., I. KIFOR, et al. 2000. Aldosterone: a mediator of myocardial necrosis and renal arteriopathy. Endocrinology **141**: 3871–3878.
40. FIEBELER, A., F. SCHMIDT, D.N. MULLER, et al. 2001. Mineralocorticoid receptor affects AP-1 and nuclear factor-kappab activation in angiotensin II-induced cardiac injury. Hypertension 37 (2 Part 2): 787–793.
41. FRIEDMAN, S.M. & C.L. FRIEDMAN. 1948 Observations on the role of the rat kidney in hypertension caused by deoxycorticosterone acetate. J. Exp. Med.: **87**: 329.

42. SELYE, H. 1946. The general adaptation syndrome and the diseases of adaptation. J. Clin. Endocrinol. **6:** 117–230.
43. ROCHA, R., A.E. RUDOLPH, G.E. FRIERDICH, *et al.* 2002. Aldosterone induces a vascular inflammatory phenotype in the rat heart. Am. J. Physiol. Heart Circ. Physiol. **283:** in press.
44. SABBAH, H.N., G. SUZUKI, H. MORITA, *et al.* 2002. Eplerenone, a novel aldosterone receptor antagonist, prevents progressive left ventricular dysfunction and attenuates remodeling in dogs with heart failure. Presented at the 66th Annual Scientific Meeting of the Japanese Circulation Society, Sapporo, Japan, April 26 .
45. GOMEZ-SANCHEZ, E.P., M.T. VENKATARAMAN, D. THWAITES & C. FORT. 1990. ICV infusion of corticosterone antagonizes ICV-aldosterone hypertension. Am. J. Physiol. **258** (4 Pt 1)**:** E649–653.
46. SAKAI, R.R., B.S. MCEWEN, S.J. FLUHARTY & L.Y. MA. 2000. Amygdala: site of genomic and nongenomic arousal of aldosterone-induced sodium intake. Kidney Int. **57:** 1337–1345.
47. ROCHA, R. & C.T. STIER. 2002. Role of aldosterone in the development of stroke in genetically hypertensive rats. Presented at the 66th Annual Meeting of the Japanese Circulation Society, Sapporo, Japan, April 24.
48. ROCHA, R., P.N CHANDER, K. KHANNA, *et al.* 1998. Mineralocorticoid blockade reduces vascular injury in stroke-prone hypertensive rats. Hypertension. **31** (1 Pt 2)**:** 451–458.
49. ROCHA, R., P.N. CHANDER, A. ZUCKERMAN, *et al.* 1999. Role of aldosterone in renal vascular injury in stroke-prone hypertensive rats. Hypertension. **33** (1 Pt 2)**:** 232–237.
50. WEBER, K.T. 2001. Aldosterone in congestive heart failure. N. Engl. J. Med. **345:** 1689–1697.

Familial/Sporadic Glucocorticoid Resistance Syndrome and Hypertension

TOMOSHIGE KINO, ALESSANDRA VOTTERO,
EVANGELIA CHARMANDARI, AND GEORGE P. CHROUSOS

Pediatric and Reproductive Endocrinology Branch, National Institute of Child Health and Human Development, National Institutes of Health, Bethesda, Maryland 20892, USA

ABSTRACT: Glucocorticoids regulate diverse functions important for the maintenance of central nervous system, cardiovascular, metabolic, and immune homeostasis. The actions of these hormones are mediated by the specific intracellular glucocorticoid receptors (GRs). Pathologic conditions associated with changes of tissue sensitivity to these hormones have been described. The syndrome of familial/sporadic glucocorticoid resistance is characterized by hypercortisolism without Cushing syndrome stigmata. Many of the patients present with hypertension, with or without hypokalemic alkalosis, as a result of elevated concentrations of cortisol and other salt-retaining steroids. The molecular defects of 4 kindreds and one sporadic case have been elucidated as inactivating mutations in the ligand-binding domain of the GR. In two patients in whom the GR was mutated at amino acid isoleucine 559 to aspartic acid (GRαI559N) and isoleucine 747 to methionine (GRαI747M), respectively, glucocorticoid resistance developed at the heterozygous state, with transdominant negative activity of each of the mutant receptors upon the wild-type protein. Retention of the wild-type receptor in the cytoplasm by the mutant receptor was found in the former, while inappropriate accumulation of p160-type coactivators on the promoter region of glucocorticoid-responsive genes, because of a defective interaction between the AF2 region of the mutant receptor and the LXXLL motif of the coactivators, was determined in the latter. These results suggest that the pathologic mechanisms of glucocorticoid resistance is quite broad, and this is reflected in the wide variability of the clinical picture in patients with the syndrome.

KEYWORDS: glucocorticoid receptor; tissue sensitivity to glucocorticoids; mutation; nuclear translocation; p160 coactivators

INTRODUCTION

The glucocorticoids exert profound influences on many physiologic functions by virtue of their diverse roles in growth, development, and maintenance of homeostasis.[1,2] The action of glucocorticoids are mediated by the intracellular glucocorticoid receptor (GR), which functions as a hormone-activated transcription factor that regulates the expression of glucocorticoid target genes.[3] The GR is ubiquitously expressed in almost all human tissues and organs. The presence of glucocorticoids is crucial for the integrity of central nervous system (CNS) function and for maintenance of cardiovascular, metabolic and immune homeostasis.[4] Increased glucocorticoid secretion during stress alters CNS function, assists with adjustments in energy expenditures and modulates the inflammatory/immune response.[4] The potent immunosuppressive effects of glucocorticoids also make them indispensable therapeutic compounds for many inflammatory, autoimmune and lymphoproliferative diseases. Thus, change of tissue sensitivity to glucocorticoids may not only lead to numerous pathologic conditions but also it may influence the outcome of therapeutic intervention with glucocorticoids.

There are two opposite directions in the change of tissue sensitivity to glucocorticoids: *glucocorticoid resistance* and *hypersensitivity*. Several pathologic conditions are known to and/or associated with such diametrically opposed changes, for example, familial/sporadic generalized glucocorticoid resistance, several autoimmune and inflammatory diseases, such as rheumatoid arthritis and glucocorticoid resistant asthma, are known as examples of the former condition, while visceral obesity-related insulin resistance/hypertension and acquired immunodeficiency syndrome caused by human immunodeficiency virus type-1 infection have been related to the latter.[5,6]

The syndrome of familial/sporadic glucocorticoid resistance is the most well-examined pathologic condition, associated with altered tissue sensitivity to glucocorticoids. Since glucocorticoids possess a broad array of life-sustaining functions, only patients with partial or incomplete glucocorticoid resistance have been reported so far, suggesting that complete inability of glucocorticoids to exert their effects on their target tissues are incompatible with human life.[5] More than 10 kindreds and individual patients suffering from congenital glucocorticoid resistance have been described to date and the molecular mechanisms of their resistance have been analyzed in some of them.[4,7,8]

STRUCTURE AND FUNCTIONS OF THE GLUCOCORTICOID RECEPTOR

The glucocorticoid receptor (GR) is a member of the steroid/sterol/thyroid/retinoid/orphan receptor superfamily of nuclear transactivating factors, with more than 150 members currently cloned and characterized across species.[9] Together with the progesterone, estrogen, androgen and mineralocorticoid receptors, the GR forms the steroid receptor subfamily. Steroid receptors display a modular structure comprising five to six regions (A–F), with the N-terminal A/B region harboring an autonomous activation function (activation function 1, AF1), and the C and E regions corresponding to the DNA- and ligand-binding domains (FIG. 1). The human GR consists of 777 amino acids, and shares similar DNA-binding domain (DBD) and closely related ligand-binding domain (LBD), but a divergent N-terminal A/B region, with other members of steroid receptor subfamily.[7]

The GR in the unliganded state is located primarily in the cytoplasm, as part of hetero-oligomeric complexes containing heat shock proteins 90, 70 and 50, and, possibly, other proteins.[3] After binding to its ligand, the GR undergoes conformational changes, dissociates from the heat shock proteins, homodimerizes, and translocates into the nucleus, where it interacts with hormone-responsive elements and/or other transcription factors in the promoter regions of target genes.[10] The GR contains two nuclear translocation signals (NL) 1 and 2. The former is located in the boundary of DBD and the hinge region of the LBD, while the latter spans almost the entire LBD. The NL1 activity is mediated by the classic nuclear translocation system through the nuclear pore, catalyzed by importin α/β.[11]

The GR binds to and modulates transcription driven by the glucocorticoid-responsive element (GRE)-containing murine mammary tumor virus (MMTV) promoter and other active endogenous GREs, which are present in the promoter regions of many glucocorticoid-responsive genes. Concerted stimulation of transcription by AF1 and 2 is required for the full activation of target promoters. AF2, which is formed by helices 3, 4 and 12 of the LBD, attracts coactivators such as p300 and its homologous protein, CREB-binding protein (CBP), p160-type coactivators, and p300/CBP-associated protein (p/CAF).[12] Helix 12 of the LBD plays a pivotal role in the formation of the AF2 surface, by changing its position in response to ligands. AF2 directly binds coactivators through their LXXLL coactivator motifs, where L is leucine and X is any amino acids.[13] The mechanism of transcriptional activation by AF1 is not well known, but p160 coactivators and the newly identified riboprotein steroid receptor coactivator (SRA) also contribute to its activity.[12] The GR as a dimer/monomer also modulates the transcription rates of non-GRE-containing genes, which are regulated by other transcription factors, such as AP-1,[14] NF-κB,[15] and STAT5,[16] through protein–protein interactions with these factors.

The human GR cDNA was isolated by expression cloning in 1985.[17] The genes of the GR consists of 9 exons; its locus is on chromosome 5 (FIG. 1). There are two 3′ splicing variants, GRα and β, from alternative use of a different terminal exon 9α or 9β. GRα is the classic GR that binds with gluco-

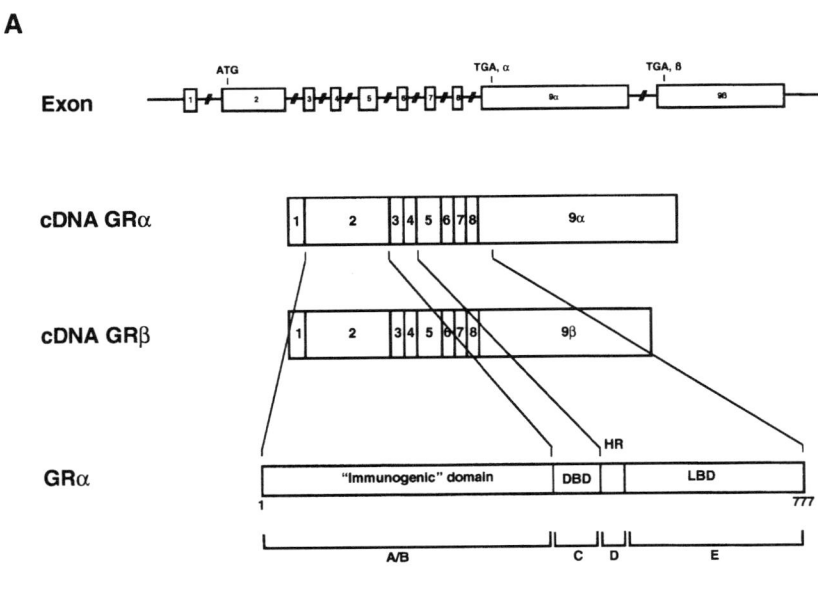

FIGURE 1. (**A** and **B**) Genomic structure and domains of linearized GRα and GRβ molecules. GR = glucocorticoid receptor; HR = hinge region; DBD = DNA-binding domain; LBD = ligand-binding domain; NL = nuclear localization signal; AF1 and AF2 = activation function 1 and 2.

corticoids and transactivates or transrepresses glucocorticoid-responsive promoters. On the other hand, GRβ does not bind glucocorticoids and functions as a weak dominant negative inhibitor of GRα on GRE-containing, glucocorticoid-responsive promoters.[18]

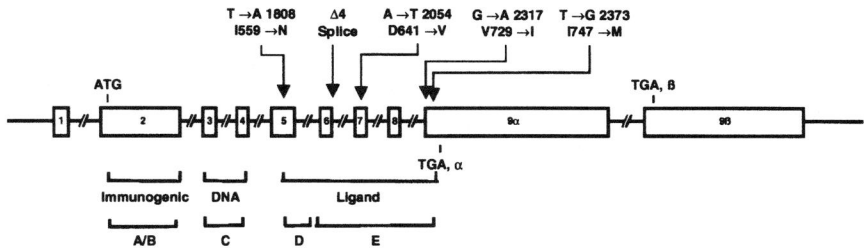

FIGURE 2. Location of the known mutations of the glucocorticoid receptor in its genomic structures.

HORMONE RESISTANCE CAUSED BY MUTATIONS IN THE GLUCOCORTICOID RECEPTOR GENE: GLUCOCORTICOID RECEPTOR MUTATIONS

The syndrome of familiar/sporadic glucocorticoid resistance, first described in 1976, is a disorder characterized by hypercorticosolism without Cushingoid features.[19,20] Since then, more than 10 kindreds and sporadic cases have been reported.[21–29] Abnormalities of the GR number, affinity for glucocorticoids, stability, and translocation into the nucleus have been described. The molecular defects of 4 kindreds and one sporadic case have been elucidated so far (FIG. 2; TABLE 1). The propositus of the original kindred was found by Hurley et al. to be a homozygote for a single nonconservative point mutation, replacing aspartic acid with valine at amino acid 641 in the LBD of the GR; this mutation reduced binding affinity for dexamethasone by threefold and caused loss of transactivation activity on the MMTV promoter.[26] The proposita of the second family had 4-base deletion at 3′-boundary of exon 6, removing a donor splice site. This resulted in complete ablation of one of the GR alleles in affected members of the family.[27] The propositus of the third kindred had a single homozygotic point mutation at amino acid 729 (valine to isoleucine) in the hormone binding domain, which reduced both the affinity and transactivation activity of the GR.[28] There was also an interesting sporadic case of a man with a *de novo*, germ-line, heterozygotic GR mutation at amino acid 559 (isoleucin to asparagine) in the LBD at the hinge region, close to NL1. This mutant GR had virtually no ligand-binding activity but exerted dominant negative activity upon the wild-type receptor.[29] It is present in the cytoplasm in the absence of ligand and slowly enters the nucleus in response to very high concentration of glucocorticoids after prolonged exposure. When it is coexpressed with the wild-type receptor, it delays

TABLE 1. Mutations of the GR causing glucocorticoid resistance

Author	Mutation Position cDNA	Amino Acid	Localization	Biochemical Phenotype	Genotype/Transmission
Hurley et al.[26]	2054(A→T)	641(D→V)	E	Affinity↓ Transactivation↓	Homozygote/autosomal recessive
Karl et al.[27]	Δ4 at the 3′ boundary of exon and intron 6		E	Number↓ Inactivation of the affected allele	Heterozygote/autosomal dominant
Malchoff et al.[28]	2317(G→A)	729(V→I)	E	Affinity↓ Transactivation↓	Homozygote/autosomal recessive
Karl et al.[29]	1808(T→A)	559(I→N)	D	Number↓ Transactivation↓ Dominant negative activity on wild type	Heterozygote/ sporadic
Vottero et al.[31]	2373(T→G)	747(I→M)	E	Affinity↓ Transactivation↓ Dominant negative activity on wild type	Heterozygote/autosomal dominant

translocation of the wild-type receptor into the cytoplasm, which explains its dominant negative activity upon the wild-type receptor.[30]

Recently, study of a fifth case/kindred with glucocorticoid resistance and a heterozygotic GR mutation in the LBD (amino acid 747, replacing isoleucine with methionine) was determined; the mutant receptor had mildly reduced affinity for dexamethasone and markedly decreased transactivational activity; interestingly, it also had dominant negative activity upon the wild-type receptor.[31] The mutation is located just several amino acids prior to the helix 12 of the LBD, which plays a pivotal role in the formation of the AF2 of the ligand-activated GR. This mutant receptor cannot bind to the nuclear coactivator signature motif, LXXLL, of the p160-type nuclear receptor coactivators but continues to associate with this type of coactivator through its intact AF1 domain located in the N-terminal immunogenic domain. Overexpression of p160 coactivators diminished the dominant negative activity of the mutant receptor. This suggests that defective interaction of the mutant receptor with p160 coactivators may explain its dominant negative activity on the wild-type receptor, possibly by the formations of ineffective coactivator complexes on the promoter region of target genes.[31]

PATHOPHYSIOLOGY OF FAMILIAL GLUCOCORTICOID RESISTANCE

A complex negative feedback system exists in the human CNS that regulates glucocorticoid homeostasis. Glucocorticoids exert negative feedback effects on both the hypothalamic corticotropin-releasing hormone (CRH) and arginine vasopressin (AVP) secretion and inhibit pituitary ACTH production and secretion itself. In addition, glucocorticoids influence the activity of suprahypothalamic centers that control the activity of CRH and AVP neurons.[4] This complex regulatory system is activated in patients with loss-of-function GR mutations, resulting in compensatory increases in ACTH and cortisol secretion (FIG. 3). The patients retain the circadian rhythm and responsiveness of cortisol to stress, but are resistant to single or multiple doses of dexamethasone.

Although adequate compensation is apparently achieved by elevated cortisol concentrations in the great majority of the patients described, excess ACTH secretion also results in increased production of adrenal steroids with mineralocorticoid activity and enhanced secretion of adrenal androgens. The former, together with cortisol, is responsible for causing symptoms and signs of mineralocorticoid excess, such as hypertension and/or hypokalemic alkalosis, whereas the latter causes varying manifestations of hyperandrogenism, such as acne, hirsutism, male pattern baldness, menstrual irregularities and infertility in women. Precocious puberty has been seen in a child due to early

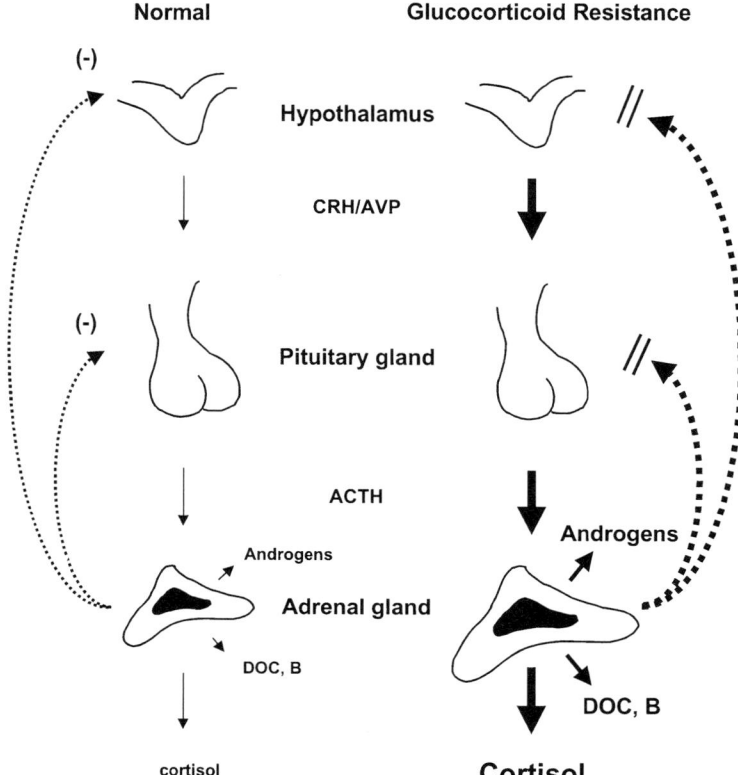

FIGURE 3. Pathophysiologic mechanism of glucocorticoid resistance induced by loss-of-function GR mutations. The elaborate negative feedback mechanism responsible for maintenance of glucocorticoid homeostasis compensates for tissue insensitivity to glucocorticoids by resetting the hypothalamic-pituitary-adrenal (HPA) axis at higher level. Thus, CRH/AVP, ACTH, and cortisol secretion are increased. The compensatory increase in ACTH production augments the secretion of cortisol and glucocorticoid precursors with mineralocorticoid activity (DOC, deoxycorticosterone; B, cortisosterone), as well as the secretion of several adrenal androgens, including Δ4-androstenedione, which has considerable androgen activity.

and excessive prepubertal adrenal androgen secretion. In the male, oligospermia and infertility have been observed, possibly as a result of disturbances in FSH regulation caused by excessive adrenal androgens. However, the spectrum of clinical manifestations in patients with GR mutations is quite broad, as a large number of subjects are asymptomatic, showing only biochemical changes.

TREATMENT OF PATIENTS WITH FAMILIAL GLUCOCORTICOID RESISTANCE

Patients are treated with high doses of mineralocorticoid-sparing synthetic glucocorticoids. The goal is to suppress the increased levels of ACTH, which causes overproduction of mineralocorticoids and androgens (FIG. 3). As all cases described thus far have had partial inactivation of GR activity, synthetic potent glucocorticoids with minimal intrinsic mineralocorticoid activity, such as dexamethasone, is a rational approach. These steroids achieve activation of the mutated glucocorticoid receptor in homozygous cases or of the wild-type receptor in heterozygous cases that is sufficient to suppress the compensatory increases of ACTH, and hence the adrenal mineralocorticoid and androgen excess that cause the clinical manifestations of the condition. The patients should be treated with high, individualized doses of oral dexamethasone, which would be pharmacologic for the normal population (1–3 mg/day). Dexamethasone indeed suppresses ACTH and therefore endogenous cortisol, DOC, corticosterone and adrenal androgen secretion, correcting the mineralocorticoid and androgen excess states of these patients.

REFERENCES

1. CLARK, J.K. et al. 1992. Mechanism of steroid hormones. In Williams' Textbook of Endocrinology. J.D.Wilson, & D.W. Foster, Eds.: 35–90. W.B. Saunders Co. Philadephia, PA.
2. MUNCK, A. et al. 1984. Physiological functions of glucocorticoids in stress and their relation to pharmacological actions. Endocr. Rev. **5:** 25–44.
3. BEATO, M. & A. SANCHEZ-PACHECO. 1996. Interaction of steroid hormone receptors with the transcription initiation complex. Endocr. Rev. **17:** 587–609.
4. CHROUSOS, G.P. 1995. The hypothalamic-pituitary-adrenal axis and immune-mediated inflammation. N. Engl. J. Med. **332:** 1351–1362.
5. CHROUSOS, G.P. et al. 1993. Syndromes of glucocorticoid resistance. Ann. Intern. Med. **119:** 1113–1124.
6. KINO, T. & G.P/ CHROUSOS. 2001. Glucocorticoid and mineralocorticoid resistance/hypersensitivity syndromes. J. Endocrinol. **169:** 437–445.
7. ARAI, K. & G.P. CHROUSOS. 1995. Syndromes of glucocorticoid and mineralocorticoid resistance. Steroids **60:** 173–179.
8. DE CASTRO, M. & G.P. CHROUSOS. 1997. Glucocorticoid resistance. Curr. Ther. Endocrinol. Metab. **6:** 188–189.
9. MANGELSDORF, D.J. et al. 1995. The nuclear receptor superfamily: the second decade. Cell **83:** 835–839.
10. BAMBERGER, C.M. et al. 1996. Molecular determinants of glucocorticoid receptor function and tissue sensitivity to glucocorticoids. Endocr. Rev. **17:** 245–261.

11. SAVORY, J.G. *et al.* 1999. Discrimination between NL1- and NL2-mediated nuclear localization of the glucocorticoid receptor. Mol. Cell. Biol. **19:** 1025–1037.
12. MCKENNA, N.J. *et al.* 1999. Nuclear receptor coregulators: cellular and molecular biology. Endocr. Rev. **20:** 321–344.
13. SHIAU, A.K. *et al.* 1998. The structural basis of estrogen receptor/coactivator recognition and the antagonism of this interaction by tamoxifen. Cell **95:** 927–937.
14. SCHULE, R. *et al.* 1990. Functional antagonism between oncoprotein c-Jun and the glucocorticoid receptor. Cell **62:** 1217–1226.
15. CALDENHOVEN, E. *et al.* 1995. Negative cross-talk between RelA and the glucocorticoid receptor: a possible mechanism for the antiinflammatory action of glucocorticoids. Mol. Endocrinol. **9:** 401–412.
16. STOCKLIN, E. *et al.* 1996. Functional interactions between Stat5 and the glucocorticoid receptor. Nature **383:** 726–728.
17. HOLLENBERG, S.M. *et al.* 1985. Primary structure and expression of a functional human glucocorticoid receptor cDNA. Nature **318:** 635–641.
18. BAMBERGER, C.M. *et al.* 1995. Glucocorticoid receptor beta, a potential endogenous inhibitor of glucocorticoid action in humans. J. Clin. Invest. **95:** 2435–2441.
19. VINGERHOEDS, A.C.M. *et al.* 1976. Spontaneous hypercortisolism without Cushing's syndrome. J. Clin. Endocrinol. Metab. **43:** 1128–1133.
20. CHROUSOS, G.P. *et al.* 1982. Primary cortisol resistance in man: a glucocorticoid receptor-mediated disease. J. Clin. Invest. **69:** 1261–1269.
21. LAMBERTS, S.W. *et al.* 1986. Familial cortisol resistance: differential diagnostic and therapeutic aspects. J. Clin. Endocrinol. Metab. **63:** 1328–1333.
22. NAWATA, H. *et al.* 1987. Decreased deoxyribonucleic acid binding of glucocorticoid-receptor complex in cultured skin fibroblasts from a patient with the glucocorticoid resistance syndrome. J. Clin. Endocrinol. Metab. **65:** 219–226.
23. IIDA, S. *et al.* 1985. Primary cortisol resistance accompanied by a reduction in glucocorticoid receptors in two members of the same family. J. Clin. Endocrinol. Metab. **60:** 967–971.
24. VECSEI, P. *et al.* 1989. Primary glucocorticoid receptor defect with likely familial involvement. Cancer Res. **49:** 2220s–2221s.
25. LAMBERTS, S.W. *et al.* 1992. Cortisol receptor resistance: the variability of its clinical presentation and response to treatment. J. Clin. Endocrinol. Metab. **74:** 313–321.
26. HURLEY, D.M. *et al.* 1991. Point mutation causing a single amino acid substitution in the hormone binding domain of the glucocorticoid receptor in familial glucocorticoid resistance. J. Clin. Invest. **87:** 680–686.
27. KARL, M. *et al.* 1993. Familial glucocorticoid resistance caused by a splice site deletion in the human glucocorticoid receptor gene. J. Clin. Endocrinol. Metab. **76:** 683–689.
28. MALCHOFF, D.M. *et al.* 1993. A mutation of the glucocorticoid receptor in primary cortisol resistance. J. Clin. Invest. **91:** 1918–1925.
29. KARL, M. *et al.* 1996. Cushing's disease preceded by generalized glucocorticoid resistance: clinical consequences of a novel, dominant-negative glucocorticoid receptor mutation. Proc. Assoc. Am. Physicians **108:** 296–307.

30. KINO, T. *et al.* 2001. Pathologic human GR mutant has a transdominant negative effect on the wild-type GR by inhibiting Its translocation into the nucleus: importance of the ligand-binding domain for intracellular GR trafficking. J. Clin. Endocrinol. Metab. **86:** 5600–5608.
31. VOTTERO, A. *et al.* 2002. A novel, C-terminal dominant negative mutation of the GR causes familial glucocorticoid resistance through abnormal interactions with p160 steroid receptor coactivators. J. Clin. Endocrinol. Metab. **87:** 2658–2667.

Diagnostic Tests for Cushing's Syndrome

LYNNETTE K. NIEMAN

Pediatric and Reproductive Endocrinology Branch, National Institute of Child Health and Human Development, NIH, Bethesda, Maryland, USA

ABSTRACT: The diagnosis of Cushing's syndrome rests on the demonstration of clinical features and biochemical abnormalities that reflect hypercortisolism. If a patient presents with typical clinical features such as weight gain with truncal obesity and supraclavicular fat deposition, wide purple striae, and proximal muscle weakness, the diagnosis is clear-cut and is nearly always substantiated by a 24-hour urine free cortisol excretion value more than four times the normal level. However, many patients present with signs and symptoms that are common in the general population, such as hypertension, generalized weight gain, reproductive abnormalities, and depression. Many of these patients have normal cortisol excretion and do not have Cushing's syndrome. Others have mild hypercortisolism caused by psychiatric disorders, obligate exercise, morbid obesity, sleep apnea, or uncontrolled diabetes mellitus. These patients may be confused with those with the true Cushing's syndrome, and thus are considered to have a "pseudo-Cushing" state. Additional observation over time, and testing with midnight cortisol measurements, the 2-day–2-mg dexamethasone suppression test, or the dexamethasone suppression–CRH stimulation test may be useful to identify true Cushing's syndrome in these patients.

KEYWORDS: cortisol; ACTH; Cushing's syndrome

CLINICAL FEATURES OF CUSHING'S SYNDROME

Cushing's syndrome is a symptom complex that reflects excessive tissue exposure to cortisol. Thus, in general, patients should be screened for hypercortisolism when they present with typical signs or symptoms of the disorder.[1–4] As shown in TABLE 1, these clinical features are variable and no single pattern is seen in all patients. Also, since clinical abnormalities reflect the amount and duration of hypercortisolism, patients with mild or intermittent cortisol excess usually have fewer features than those with very high gluco-

---

Address for correspondence; Lynette K. Nieman, M.D., Building 10 Room 9D42 MSC 1583, 10 Center Drive, Bethesda, MD 20892-1583. Voice: 301-496-8935; fax: 301-402-0884.
NiemanL@nih.gov

TABLE 1. Frequency of clinical signs and symptoms of Cushing's syndrome[a]

Sign/Symptom	Percentage of 70
Decreased libido in men and women	100
Obesity or weight gain	97
Plethora	94
Round face	88
Menstrual changes	84
Hirsutism	81
Hypertension	74
Ecchymoses	62
Lethargy, depression	62
Striae	56
Weakness	56
EKG changes or atherosclerosis	55
Dorsal fat pad	54
Edema	50
Abnormal glucose tolerance	50
Osteopenia or fracture	50
Headache	47
Backache	43
Recurrent infections	25
Abdominal pain	21
Acne	21
Female balding	13

[a]Abstracted from Plotz, Knowlton, and Ragan.[1]

corticoid production. Because obesity, hypertension, menstrual irregularities, hirsutism and depression are common in patients without Cushing's syndrome, they do not predict well the presence of the disorder. In these patients with less-specific symptoms, it is useful to assess changes in mood and cognition, which may not be recognized as markers of hypercortisolism. These include decreased libido, insomnia, anxiety, decreased concentration, impaired memory (especially for recent events), and changes in appetite. Irritability, expressed as a decreased threshold for uncontrollable verbal outbursts, is often an early symptom. Clinicians may test for serial 7 subtractions and recall of three cities (or three objects) to quantify this symptom complex.[5]

As Cushing's syndrome tends to progress to ever-worsening hypercortisolism, patients often will show an increasing number of features if they are observed over time. Evaluation of old photographs for changes in facial contours and plethora may be helpful in documenting such a change.

A complicating factor in the clinical assessment of possible hypercortisolism is that few signs or symptoms are specific to Cushing's syndrome, but rather occur frequently in the general population. Hypertension illustrates this difficulty, as it is common in middle-aged or older adults, but is caused by Cushing's syndrome in very few of them. Cushing's syndrome (and other endocrine causes of hypertension) is more common in patients in whom hypertension is unusual—such as children, or in patients who have difficult in controlling hypertension, or hypertension with hypokalemia. (See the related chapter on ectopic ACTH secretion and hypertension in this volume.)

The fact that Cushing's syndrome is rare but that many of its clinical features are common in the general population raises the dilemma of who should be screened for the disorder.[4,6] Patients with minimal features, such as simple obesity alone, are unlikely to have Cushing's syndrome, and may be observed for the development of additional features over time. Such a change may increase the probability of disease, so that it may be fruitful to screen a patient with progressive clinical features. At the other end of the spectrum, patients with signs that are most characteristic of glucocorticoid excess should be screened, as the disorder is more likely in such a patient. Features most specific to Cushing's syndrome include abnormal fat distribution, particularly in the supraclavicular and temporal fossae, proximal muscle weakness, wide (>1 cm) purple striae, and decreased linear growth with continued weight gain in a child. It is also reasonable to screen patients with unexplained or unusual features for their age group, such as non-traumatic fracture in young individuals with no risk for osteopenia, and hypertension or cutaneous atrophy in young individuals. Of course, such screening would be done in the context of evaluation for other etiologic factors.

BIOCHEMICAL SCREENING TESTS FOR CUSHING'S SYNDROME

Urine Free Cortisol (UFC)

Measurement of 24-hour excretion of cortisol is the gold standard test for the diagnosis of Cushing's syndrome.[7,8] Recently many laboratories began to offer high-pressure liquid chromatography (HPLC) measurement of urine cortisol. In contrast to antibody-based assays, this method has virtually no cross-reactivity with other steroids or cortisol metabolites. As a result, the normal range is lower than that of antibody-based methods. Thus it is very important to know the assay reference range when evaluating UFC results. Values more than 4-fold the upper of normal are virtually diagnostic for Cushing's syndrome. However, UFC may be up to 4-fold increased in pseudo-Cushing's states, characterized by mild overactivation of the hypothalamic-pituitary-adrenal axis without true Cushing's syndrome. This includes certain psychiatric disorders (depression, anxiety disorder, obsessive-compulsive disorder), morbid obesity, poorly controlled diabetes mellitus, obligate exercise, sleep apnea, and alcoholism. Mildly elevated UFC also may be seen without any associated condition.[9] UFC may be falsely negative in the inactive phase of cyclic or intermittent Cushing's syndrome, and is low in severe renal failure. The test is not reliable when creatinine clearance is less than 20 cc/minute.

Because over- or under-collection may result in falsely increased or decreased results, evaluation of the total specimen volume and creatinine excretion helps to assess whether this is a concern. Creatinine excretion is relatively stable in most individuals, varying by no more than 15% from day to day.

Dexamethasone Suppression Tests

The 1-mg overnight dexamethasone suppression test (DST) is a simple screening test.[9,10] The patient takes dexamethasone, 1 mg orally, between 11 PM and midnight and reports between 8 and 9 AM the following morning for measurement of plasma cortisol. The appropriate cut-point for normal cortisol suppression is debated; a cortisol concentration of 3.6 µg/dL or less achieves high sensitivity (2% false-negative rate). There is up to 30% false-positive rate in chronic illness, obesity, psychiatric disorders, and even normal individuals[9] and false results may occur because of abnormal dexamethasone clearance.

The more cumbersome 2-mg–2-day test ("low-dose DST") also has a high false-positive rate,[9,11] using urine outcome measures, but a high sensitivity and specificity using a cortisol criterion.[10,11] If the patient can comply with the rigid scheduling requirements of dexamethasone administration, 500 mg every six hours, and the subsequent plasma cortisol collection, this can be a very useful test.

The dexamethasone–CRH stimulation test distinguishes patients with pseudo-Cushing's syndrome from those with Cushing's syndrome.[11] The test is performed by giving dexamethasone, 0.5 mg, orally every six hours for 8 doses beginning at noon, and ending at 6 AM. CRH, 1 µg/kg body weight, is given intravenously two hours after the last dose, and cortisol is measured just before CRH administration and 15 minutes later. One may measure a plasma dexamethasone level just before CRH is given to verify normal metabolism, as commercial laboratories offer this assay with the expected range of results. A plasma cortisol of ≥ 1.4 µg/dL supports the diagnosis of Cushing's syndrome, while lower values are seen in normal individuals and those with pseudo-Cushing states.

CRH is available commercially (ACTHREL®, Ferring Corp.) with FDA-approved labeling for the differential diagnosis of Cushing's syndrome. Use of the agent in the dexamethasone-CRH test represents an off-label use. Only about 100 patients have been reported using the test.[11]

Any dexamethasone test may give either false-positive or false-negative results in conditions that alter the metabolic clearance of the agent. Alcohol, rifampin, phenytoin, and phenobarbital induce the cytochrome P450-related enzymes and enhance dexamethasone clearance, while renal or hepatic failure retard dexamethasone clearance. Stop these medications if possible, or measure dexamethasone to determine whether its clearance has been altered.

Midnight Cortisol Values

Measurement of plasma cortisol at midnight through an indwelling intravenous line distinguishes pseudo-Cushing states from Cushing's syndrome, with 95% diagnostic accuracy using a cut-point of >7.5 ug/dL to diagnose Cushing's syndrome.[12] Preservation of the physiologic circadian rhythmicity of cortisol secretion in pseudo-Cushing states compared to Cushing's syndrome underlies this test.[13] Thus, patients who do not normally sleep at night and those arriving from other time zones may have abnormal results. Overall, the test has a 5% false-negative rate (usually in patients with intermittent or mild Cushing's syndrome). Others have measured midnight cortisol in blood obtained from sleeping subjects by direct venipuncture. In that study, normal individuals had a cortisol of less than 50 mmol/L, but pseudo-Cushing's syndrome patients were not evaluated.[14]

Although the dexamethasone–CRH test and midnight plasma cortisol test have a high diagnostic accuracy, they are limited by inconvenience and/or cost. Recent research at the NIH and in Milwaukee indicates that measurement of salivary cortisol at bedtime or midnight works as well as the midnight plasma cortisol test.[15,16] However, the cut-points used in the two studies are different, suggesting that the assays are different, so that salivary cortisol assays may need local validation before they are used for this purpose.

SUMMARY

The clinical diagnosis of Cushing's syndrome is straightforward if classical features—increased supraclavicular fat, truncal obesity, proximal muscle weakness, and wide purple striae—are present. Similarly, the biochemical diagnosis is secure if UFC is more than 4-fold normal in the presence of clinical signs and symptoms of Cushing's syndrome. Unfortunately, many patients have less-distinctive clinical and biochemical signs of hypercortisolism. In these individuals, causes of pseudo-Cushing states should be sought and treated, in which case hypercortisolism may remit. As shown in FIGURE 1,

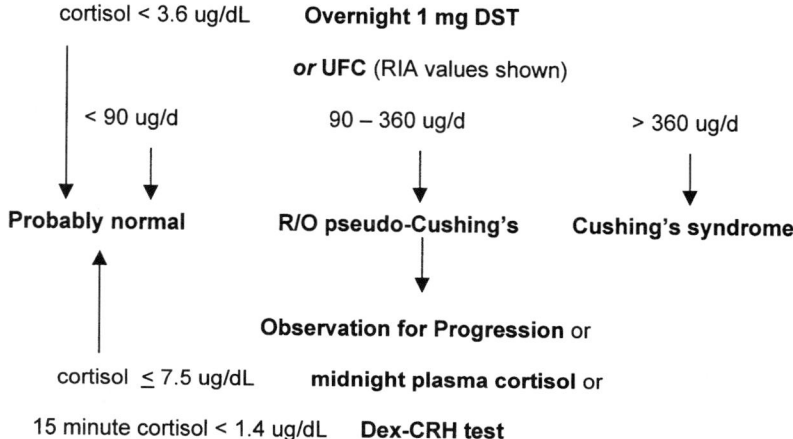

FIGURE 1. An algorithm for the diagnosis of Cushing's syndrome.

continued observation for progression of Cushingoid signs and symptoms and the use of adjunctive tests such as midnight cortisol or the dexamethasone suppression test (with or without CRH) may be helpful when the diagnosis is not clear-cut.

REFERENCES

1. PLOTZ, C.M., A.I. KNOWLTON & C. RAGAN. 1952. The natural history of Cushing's syndrome. Am. J. Med. **13:** 597–614.
2. ROSS, E.J. & D.C. LINCH. 1982. Cushing's syndrome–killing disease: discriminatory value of signs and symptoms aiding early diagnosis. Lancet **2:** 646–649.
3. SOFFER, L.J., A. IANNACCONE & I.L. GABRILOVE. 1961. Cushing's syndrome: a study of fifty patients. Am. J. Med. **300:** 129–135.
4. NIEMAN, L.K. 2000. Cushing syndrome. *In* DeGroot's Textbook of Endocrinology. W.B. Saunders. Philadelphia, PA.
5. STARKMAN, M.N., D.E. SCHTEINGART & M.A. SCHORK. 1986. Correlation of bedside cognitive and neuropsychological tests in patients with Cushing's syndrome. Psychosomatics **27:** 508–511.
6. ORTH, D. N. 1995. Cushing's syndrome. N. Engl. J. Med. **332:** 791–803.
7. MELBY, J.C. 1971. Assessment of adrenocortical function. N. Engl. J. Med. **285:** 735–739.
8. CRAPO, L. 1979. Cushing's syndrome: a review of diagnostic tests. Metabolism **28:** 955–977.
9. KAYE, T.B. & L. CRAPO. 1990. The Cushing's syndrome: an update on diagnostic tests. Ann. Intern. Med. **112:** 434–444.

10. NEWELL-PRICE, J., P. TRAINER, M. BESSER & A. GROSSMAN. 1998. The diagnosis and differential diagnosis of Cushing's syndrome and pseudo-Cushing's states. Endocr. Rev. **19:** 647–672.
11. YANOVSKI, J.A., G.B. CUTLER, JR., G.P. CHROUSOS & L.K. NIEMAN. 1993. Corticotropin-releasing hormone stimulation following low-dose dexamethasone administration: a new test to distinguish Cushing's syndrome from pseudo-Cushing's states. JAMA. **269:** 2232–2238.
12. PAPANICOLAOU, D.A., J.A. YANOVSKI, G. B. CUTLER, JR., *et al.* 1998. A single midnight serum cortisol measurement distinguishes Cushing's syndrome from pseudo-Cushing states. J. Clin. Endocrinol. Metab. **83:** 1163–1167.
13. KRIEGER, D.T., W. ALLEN, F. RIZZO & H.P. KRIEGER. 1971. Characterization of the normal temporal pattern of plasma corticosteroid levels. J. Clin. Endocrinol. Metab. **32:** 266–284.
14. NEWELL-PRICE J., P. TRAINER, L. PERRY, *et al.* 1995. A single sleeping midnight cortisol has 100% sensitivity for the diagnosis of Cushing's syndrome. Clin. Endocrinol. (Oxf.) **43:** 545–550.
15. RAFF H., J.L. RAFF & J.W. FINDLING. 1998. Late-night salivary cortisol as a screening test for Cushing's syndrome. J. Clin. Endocrinol. Metab. **83:** 2681–2686.
16. GAFNI, R.I., D.A. PAPANICOLAOU & L.K. NIEMAN. 2000. Nighttime salivary cortisol measurement as a simple, noninvasive, outpatient screening test for Cushing's syndrome in children and adolescents. J. Pediatr. **137:** 30–35.

The Medical Management of Cushing's Syndrome

DAMIAN MORRIS AND ASHLEY GROSSMAN

Department of Endocrinology, St. Bartholomew's Hospital, London EC1A 7BE, England, United Kingdom

ABSTRACT: Cushing's syndrome results from prolonged exposure to excessive circulating glucocorticosteroids, and is associated with significant morbidity and mortality. While the treatment of choice in most patients is surgical, the metabolic consequences of the syndrome, including increased tissue fragility, poor wound healing, hypertension, and diabetes mellitus, increase the risks of such surgery. The hypercortisolemia and its sequelae can be efficiently reversed using medical therapy, either as a temporary measure prior to definitive treatment, or longer term in more difficult cases. Drug treatment has been targeted at the hypothalamic/pituitary level, the adrenal glands, and also at the glucocorticoid receptor level. In this review we discuss the pharmacotherapeutic agents that have been used in Cushing's syndrome, and their efficacy, the monitoring of treatment, and potential therapies that may prove useful in the future in this complex endocrinological disorder.

KEYWORDS: Cushing's syndrome; drug therapy; steroid biosynthesis inhibitors; 5-HT antagonists; dopamine agonists; somatostatin analogues; GABA agonists; glucocorticoid antagonists

INTRODUCTION

Patients with Cushing's syndrome should have definitive treatment of the underlying cause of the hypercortisolemia if this is possible. Trans-sphenoidal surgery is the treatment of choice for pituitary-dependent Cushing's syndrome, Cushing's disease.[1] Pituitary irradiation is usually only performed when transsphenoidal surgery has failed to cure the patient. Surgical removal of an adrenocortical tumor or a source of ectopic ACTH should be the preferred treatment in patients with these diagnoses. Radiotherapy and/or che-

---

Address for correspondence: Ashley Grossman, B.A., B.Sc., M.D., FRCP, FMedSci, Professor of Neuroendocrinology, Department of Endocrinology, St. Bartholomew's Hospital, London EC1A 7BE, Great Britain. Voice: +44-(0)20-7601-8343; fax: +44-(0)20-7601-8505.
A.B.Grossman@qmul.ac.uk

motherapy may be needed for metastatic disease. However, there are numerous circumstances where medical treatment of hypercortisolemia is either desirable or essential. It is the routine practice of ourselves and other groups to pre-treat Cushing's syndrome patients prior to surgical treatment to reverse the metabolic sequelae of glucocorticoid excess, and to, it is hoped, reduce the complications of the definitive procedure. It may not always be possible to identify the source of ACTH in certain cases of ACTH-dependent Cushing's syndrome, and therefore medical management is desirable pending re-investigation. In patients in whom surgery has failed, medical management is often essential to reduce or normalize the hypercortisolemia, and should always be attempted before bilateral adrenalectomy is considered. In addition, medical treatment can be useful in patients with Cushing's disease while waiting for pituitary radiotherapy to take effect, which can take up to 10 years or more. Finally, medical therapy is helpful as a palliative modality in patients with metastatic disease causing Cushing's syndrome.

Medical therapy can be divided into three types: adrenolytic agents; neuromodulatory agents; and glucocorticoid receptor antagonists. Of these, the former are by far the most successful and therefore widely used. In this chapter we outline the drugs that have been studied and their effectiveness, and comment on possible future therapies.

ADRENOLYTIC THERAPY

Adrenolytic agents are primarily used as inhibitors of steroid biosynthesis in the adrenal cortex, and thus can be utilized in all cases of hypercortisolemia regardless of cause, often with rapid improvement in the clinical features of Cushing's syndrome. The most common agents available are metyrapone, ketoconazole, aminoglutethimide, mitotane, and etomidate.

Metyrapone

Metyrapone was introduced in 1959 as a tool for the investigation of Cushing's syndrome,[2] but has now been superseded by superior tests.[3] However, as an adrenolytic agent it continues to play an important role in the treatment of Cushing's syndrome. Metyrapone acts primarily to inhibit the enzyme 11β-hydroxylase, thus blocking the production of cortisol from 11-deoxycortisol in the adrenal gland.[4] The subsequent elevation of 11-deoxycortisol can be monitored in the serum of patients treated with metyrapone. It should be noted that there may be some cross-reactivity from 11-deoxycortisol with some cortisol radioimmunoassays: this may result in an unnecessary increase in the metyrapone dose and subsequent clinical hypoadrenalism.[5] The fall in cortisol is rapid, with trough levels at 2 hours post dose, and in our unit we usually administer a test dose of 750 mg with hourly cortisol estimation for 4 hours.[6] Maintenance therapy is in 3–4 divided doses daily.

Metyrapone has been used to good effect to reduce the hypercortisolemia in patients with Cushing's syndrome from adrenal tumors and the ectopic ACTH syndrome, either as monotherapy or in combination with aminoglutethimide[7,8] or sodium valproate,[9] although we would not recommend either of these additional agents. The effect on the clinical symptoms in these series has been variable. There has been some controversy in the past as to whether metyrapone is effective sole therapy in Cushing's disease, where it has been stated that the adrenal block is overcome by the compensatory rise in ACTH in patients not having received pituitary radiotherapy.[10] However, we and others have not found this generally to be a clinical problem.[11–13] In our series published in 1991, metyrapone was used as short-term (1–16 weeks) therapy prior to definitive treatment in 53 patients with Cushing's disease, successfully lowering mean cortisol levels to less than 400 nmol/L with dose titration.[6] While ACTH levels increased in 76% of patients, this did not have an effect on cortisol control. In addition, 30 patients with Cushing's disease received long-term metyrapone (24 after pituitary radiotherapy, and 6 without radiotherapy). In the latter group, treatment only became ineffective in three patients after 7–17 months. Therefore, this study confirms the efficacy of metyrapone in Cushing's disease, as well as in adrenocortical tumors and the ectopic ACTH syndrome. Doses required varied between 500–6000 mg/day, but were significantly less in the former two groups than the ectopic ACTH syndrome. The principal side effects with metyrapone are hirsutism and acne (as predicted by the rise in adrenal androgens), dizziness, and gastrointestinal upset. However, it is hypoadrenalism that remains the most important potential problem, and careful monitoring of treatment and education of the patient is required (*vide infra*). Hypokalemia, edema, and hypertension due to raised mineralocorticoids are infrequent,[6] but can require cessation of therapy.[14] Our experience would suggest that the only major problems are associated with the rise in adrenal androgens, which can clearly be problematic in female patients.

Ketoconazole

Ketoconazole is an imidazole derivative which was originally developed as an oral antifungal agent. However, reports of gynecomastia in some ketoconazole-treated patients led to the realization that it is an inhibitor of sex steroid production by its action on C17-20 lyase, and cortisol secretion by 11β-hydroxylase inhibition.[15–17] It also inhibits 17-hydroxylase and 18-hydroxylase activity, among other enzymes.[18] It has also been reported to have a direct effect on ectopic ACTH secretion from a thymic carcinoid tumor.[19] Treatment for Cushing's syndrome is usually started at a dose of 200 mg twice daily, and its onset of action is slower than that of metyrapone. It has been used sucessfully to lower cortisol levels in patients with Cushing's syndrome of various etiologic origins including adrenal carcinoma, the ectopic ACTH syndrome, and invasive ACTH-producing pituitary carcinoma, with doses required between 200–1200 mg/day in up to four divided daily doses.[20–25] The clinical effects of Cushing's syndrome, including hypertension, hypokalemia, and diabetes mellitus, are quick to resolve, and antihypertensives and hypoglycemic agents can often be discontinued.

The principal side effect of ketoconazole is hepatotoxicity. Reversible elevation of hepatic serum transaminases occurs in approximately 5–10% of patients, with the incidence of serious hepatic injury at around 1 in 15,000 patients.[26] Histologic changes in cases of severe hepatic injury can vary from predominantly cholestasis to extensive hepatocellular necrosis, which can be fatal or require liver transplantation.[27–29] The mean duration of treatment before the onset of jaundice is 61 days in one series, with no cases reported before 10 days.[30] The hepatotoxicity appears to be idiosyncratic, but has been reported within 7 days of the start of treatment in a patient with Cushing's syndrome,[31] although to our knowledge no resultant death in this patient group has been reported. Other adverse reactions of ketoconazole include skin rashes and gastrointestinal upset,[21] and one must always be wary of causing adrenal insufficiency.[31,32] Owing to its C17-20 lyase inhibition and consequent anti-androgenic properties, ketoconazole is particularly useful in female patients where hirsutism is an issue, which may be worsened with metyrapone. Conversely, gynecomastia and reduced libido in male patients may be unacceptable and require alternative agents. One further advantage of ketoconazole is its inhibition of cholesterol synthesis, particularly LDL cholesterol,[33] and in 34 patients with Cushing's syndrome the mean total cholesterol was reduced from 6.1 to 5.0 mmol/L on ketoconazole.[21]

Aminoglutethimide

Aminoglutethimide was introduced in 1959 as an anticonvulsant; it was noticed to induce hypothyroidism and adrenal insufficiency, and was subsequently shown to inhibit the side-chain cleavage of cholesterol to pregnenolone.[34,35] It thus inhibits not only cortisol but also estrogen and aldosterone production. In addition, it has also been shown to inhibit the enzymes 11β-hydroxylase and 18-hydroxylase, and aromatase, which converts androgens to estrogens.[36] Early reports of the use of aminoglutethimide in Cushing's syndrome showed improvement in measures of glucocorticoid production in the majority of patients.[37,39] In the largest series of 66 patients with Cushing's syndrome, reported by Misbin *et al.*,[38] a favorable response to aminoglutethimide was seen in 14 of 33 with Cushing's disease, all 6 with adrenal adenomas, 4 of 6 with the ectopic ACTH syndrome, and 13 of 21 with adrenal carcinoma. Overall, this drug seems to be less efficient at treating Cushing's disease compared to the other causes of Cushing's syndrome, which may be due to an increase in ACTH overcoming the enzymatic blockade,[39] or by hepatic enzyme induction increasing the drug's own metabolism, or a combination of both. The latter effect may also explain tolerance with continued treatment and the common side effects of rashes, fever, dizziness, and lethargy. The incidence of such adverse reactions is high, up to 58% as reported in the above series,[38] and generally limits its use.

Combination treatment with metyrapone has been used to try to reduce the dose ($\leq$750mg/day) and thus the toxicity of aminoglutethimide, and appears to be better tolerated.[8]

Mitotane

Mitotane (o,p'-DDD), an isomer of the insecticide DDD (belonging to the same family of chemicals as the insecticide DDT), was developed following the observation of adrenal atrophy in dogs administered DDD. It reduces cortisol and aldosterone production by blocking cholesterol side-chain cleavage and 11β-hydroxylase in the adrenal gland.[40]

Mitotane was introduced as a treatment for adrenal carcinoma in 1960,[41] and appears to cause tumor regression and improved survival in some patients, and has a beneficial effect on endocrine hypersecretion in approximately 75% of patients.[42] It was subsequently reported as a treatment for hypercortisolemia in Cushing's syndrome a year later.[43] In a large study of the effects of mitotane in 62 patients with Cushing's disease, of 46 patients who received mitotane alone, 38 showed remission on the basis of urinary 17-hydroxycorticosteroids at a mean of 8 months on treatment.[44] All 16 patients who received both mitotane and pituitary radiotherapy were controlled. This study highlighted the slow onset of action of mitotane, and interestingly showed that the adrenolytic effects of mitotane on biochemical remission can last for a considerable amount of time after the drug is stopped (up to 2 years). High doses of mitotane were used in this study (up to 12 g/day), similar to doses used in adrenocortical carcinoma, and consequently the incidence of adrenal insufficiency and adverse events, particularly gastrointestinal upset (57%), was high. Other side effects of mitotane include neurological disturbance, elevation of hepatic enzymes, hypercholesterolemia, hypouricemia, gynecomastia in men, and prolonged bleeding time.[42,45] Changes in hormone-binding globulins including thyroid-binding globulin also occur and total hormone measurements are unreliable during therapy.[46]

We and others have preferred a lower-dose mitotane regime as this reduces the incidence of side effects. Schteingart *et al.* used low-dose mitotane (up to 4 g/day) in combination with pituitary radiotherapy in 36 patients with Cushing's disease, and showed a remission rate of 80%. We have used similar low doses to good effect, although the onset of the cortisol-lowering effect takes longer (6–8 weeks) than with higher doses. To offset this we have used metyrapone as an adjunctive agent in the early stages, weaning this off as the mitotane takes effect.[5] One major problem even with lose-dose mitotane is the hypercholesterolemia (principally an increase in LDL-cholesterol), which appears to be due to the impairment of hepatic production of oxysterols, normally a brake on the enzyme HMG Co A reductase.[47] However, simvastatin, a HMG Co A reductase inhibitor, can reverse the hypercholesterolemia, and it or a similar agent should be used if necessary in patients treated with mitotane.[47] In the long term, measurement of blood levels should allow dose titration and reduction as appropriate.

Etomidate

Etomidate is an imidazole-derived anesthetic agent which was reported to have an adverse effect on adrenocortical function in 1983.[48] Compared to the other imidazole derivative, ketoconazole, etomidate more potently inhibits adrenocortical 11β-hydroxylase, has a similar inhibition of 17-hydroxylase, but has less of an effect on C17-20 lyase.[49] At higher concentrations it also appears to have an effect on cholesterol side-chain cleavage.[50,51]

Following their initial report in 1983,[52] Allolio *et al.* have shown that low-dose intravenous nonhypnotic etomidate (2.5 mg/hour) normalized cortisol levels in five patients with Cushing's syndrome of various etiologic origin.[53] Since then, there have been a number of case reports, including our own, on the use of mitotane in successfully reducing hypercortisolemia in seriously ill patients with either Cushing's disease or the ectopic ACTH syndrome.[54–56] We have found that a dose of etomidate of 2.5 mg/hour reducing to 1.2 mg/hour abolished endogenous cortisol production in a patient with the ectopic ACTH syndrome, but we have only been able to normalize cortisol levels in two patients with Cushing's disease, which probably reflects the increased ACTH drive from the pituitary, as opposed to relatively fixed production from an ectopic source.[55] In the latest of these reports by Krakoff *et al.*, etomidate therapy was administered intermittently over a total period of 5.5 months, usually at a dose of between 1.6–4.2 mg/hour, although during a period of recovery from hemodialysis requiring renal failure a dose of 8.3 mg/hour was required to control the hypercortisolemia.[56] Clearly, etomidate is an effective adrenolytic agent that acts rapidly, but is limited in its use by the fact it has to be given parenterally. However, in this situation it may be life-saving.

NEUROMODULATORY AGENTS

The precise mechanism of action of many of these agents is incompletely understood, although most seem to reduce ACTH secretion through an effect on the hypothalamo-pituitary axis. Their efficacy seems to be quite variable between individual patients, and overall they are much less widely used in the medical management of Cushing's syndrome than adrenolytic agents.

5-HT Antagonists

Cyproheptadine

Cyproheptadine is a histamine and serotonin (5-HT) antagonist with poor selectivity for receptor subtypes. At a dose of 24 mg/day it was shown to result in significant reduction in ACTH and prolactin levels in three of four patients with Nelson's syndrome, which led to the hypothesis that ACTH secretion is directly under a degree of serotoninergic central nervous system control.[57] Others have suggested that cyproheptadine exerts its action due to direct inhibitory effects on CRH and vasopressin secretion from the hypothalamus.[58] Support for this hypothesis comes from a study on two patients with presumed hypothalamic Cushing's disease (hyperpulsatile cortisol secretion and no adenoma on imaging), and a patient with a pituitary adenoma. In the former two patients, cyproheptadine induced biochemical and clinical remission for 3.5 and 5.5 years respectively, but had no significant effect in the patient with the adenoma.[59] In contrast, cyproheptadine was extremely effective therapy for 11 years in a patient with a resistant pituitary microadenoma.[60] However, it has also been suggested that it works independent of any neurotransmitter through a direct action on the pituitary. Thus, the usefulness of cyproheptadine in patients with Cushing's disease is extremely variable, but that it has been predicted that up to approximately 70% of patients may respond.[61] The main side effect at the usual dose of 24 mg/day is sedation. It is rarely used nowadays.

Ritanserin

Ritanserin, a specific $5-HT_2$ receptor antagonist, has also been assessed in Cushing's disease. An initial report showed a favorable response in two of three patients, after failed pituitary surgery, treated with ritanserin 10–15 mg/day for one month.[62] However, a subsequent study by the same group using ritanserin or ketanserin (a similar drug) in 11 patients with Cushing's disease, while showing a promising response to treatment in 8 patients, found that this was sustained in only 3 patients.[63]

Dopamine Agonists

Bromocriptine

This ergot derivative is a potent agonist at dopamine receptors, and has been used successfully for many years in hyperprolactinemia. Plasma ACTH levels have been shown to fall in approximately half of patients with Cushing's disease (including Nelson's syndrome) treated with a single dose of bromocriptine 2.5 mg.[64] Boscaro *et al.* studied 9 patients with Cushing's disease in an attempt to identify whether this response to a single dose of bromocriptine predicted long-term efficacy of the drug, and showed that it did not.[65] Overall, the effectiveness of long-term bromocriptine in the treatment of Cushing's disease seems quite variable,[61] and even with high doses (up to 40 mg/day) at best probably produces clinical improvement in about 50% of cases.[66] However, our own experience is that the response rate is very much less than this, and we have not seen responsivity, certainly in long-term use, in more than 1–2% of patients with Cushing's disease. Other dopamine agonists do not seem to be more effective, although one recent report has suggested that cabergoline may have significant response rates.[67] Adverse effects of bromocriptine include nasal congestion, nausea, and postural hypotension, and doses should be introduced slowly and taken in the middle of a meal. The exact mechanism of action of bromocriptine on ACTH modulation is unclear, although various hypotheses have been proposed. It has been suggested that bromocriptine responsiveness is indicative of Cushing's disease of intermediate lobe origin, as evidenced by the presence of argyrophilic fibers in these tumors.[68] In contrast, bromocriptine responsiveness has also been demonstrated in Cushing's disease due to corticotrophic hyperplasia and in an apparently normal pituitary.[69] Alternative mechanisms proposed have been through action on CRH, or a direct effect on anterior pituitary cells.[65]

Somatostatin Analogues

Octreotide

The long-acting somatostatin analogue, octreotide, is used extensively in a spectrum of neuroendocrine tumors, including somatotroph pituitary adenomas, to control hypersecretion by its action on somatostatin receptors. It has also been studied in a variety of types of Cushing's syndrome, and is effective in some patients with ACTH-dependent disease, but appears generally ineffective in adrenocortical tumors.[70] There is *in vitro* evidence of somatostatin receptor expression in corticotroph adenomas,[71] yet octreotide appears to inhibit ACTH release in Nelson's syndrome, but rarely in patients with Cushing's disease.[72] This has been postulated to be due to somatostatin receptor downregulation from the circulating hypercortisolemia.[70] Not surprisingly, many ectopic ACTH-producing tumors of neuroendocrine origin also express somatostatin receptors, and octreotide has been shown to be effective in the hypercortisolemia from such tumors.[73,74] Preoperative assessment with penetreotide scintigraphy may help predict which tumors might respond to treatment.

Octreotide may also have a role in combined therapy, as its use in combination with ketoconazole successfully normalized the hypercortisolemia in three of the four patients with Cushing's disease or the ectopic ACTH syndrome, whereas monotherapy with either agent had failed.[74]

GABA Agonists

Sodium Valproate

Sodium valproate was introduced as an anti-epileptic agent in 1978, and inhibits γ-aminobutyric acid (GABA) aminotransferase. There have been a number of reports of the effectiveness of sodium valproate to reduce ACTH levels and cause clinical remission in Cushing's disease.[75,76] In a patient with Nelson's syndrome, 600 mg of sodium valproate for 3 months significantly reduced the ACTH levels, but did not reduce the excessive ACTH response to exogenous CRH, suggesting that sodium valproate may exert its action at the hypothalamic level on CRH secretion.[77] However, a more recent study in 19 patients with Cushing's disease showed sodium valproate to be ineffective long term in all the patients studied, either as primary therapy or after failed pituitary surgery.[78]

GLUCOCORTICOID ANTAGONISTS

Mifepristone

Mifepristone (RU 486) is a potent antagonist of glucocorticoid and progesterone receptors.[79] It was developed primarily as an abortifacient. In primates and humans, mifepristone blocks glucocorticoid negative feedback at the hypothalamo-pituitary level, inducing a rise in ACTH, arginine-vasopressin (AVP), and thus cortisol.[80] This effect occurs in parallel with the normal circadian rhythm of ACTH and cortisol secretion.[81] The major drawback is the lack of biochemical markers to monitor overtreatment, and its long half-life and minimal agonist activity leaves the patient open to hypoadrenalism. In 1985 Nieman *et al.* reported clinical improvement in a patient with the ectopic ACTH syndrome treated with mifepristone at doses of up to 20 mg/kg for 9 weeks.[82] However, in a study of the short-term effects of mifepristone in seven patients with Cushing's syndrome, two patients with Cushing's disease experienced symptoms such as nausea, headache, and lethargy, which improved with high-dose intravenous dexamethasone, and therefore may have been due to hypoadrenalism.[83] Thus, while this can be useful, the drug needs to be used with great caution in Cushing's syndrome.[84]

MONITORING TREATMENT

It is important to monitor all patients on medical therapy for Cushing's syndrome, to assess the effectiveness of treatment, and in particular to avoid adrenal insufficiency. For patients on adrenolytic and neuromodulatory agents, we would advocate using the mean of five serum cortisol measurements across the day, rather than urinary free cortisol (UFC) estimations. We have shown that a mean serum cortisol between 150 to 300 nmol/L corresponds to a normal cortisol production rate,[85] and this range should be the aim of therapy. Monitoring treatment biochemically on the glucocorticoid receptor antagonist mifepristone is unhelpful (*vide supra*), and this limits it use.

FUTURE STRATEGIES

The occurrence of gastric inhibitory polypeptide (GIP)-dependent Cushing's syndrome due to abnormal expression of adrenal GIP receptors is well described,[86] but in addition patients have been described in whom cortisol production seems to be dependent on other receptors including β-adrenergic receptors, luteinizing hormone (LH) receptors, and 5-HT-4 receptors, and specific receptor antagonists may prove to be useful in such patients in the future.[87]

Retinoic acid has recently been found to inhibit ACTH secretion and cell proliferation both *in vitro* in ACTH-producing tumor cell lines, and cultured human corticotroph adenomas, and *in vivo* in nude mice.[88] This effect seems to be mediated through inhibition of the transcriptional activity of AP-1 and the orphan nuclear receptors, Nur77 and Nurr1. These potential antisecretory and antiproliferative actions of this agent in Cushing's syndrome need to be investigated further.

CONCLUSIONS

A number of drugs have been used in the medical management of Cushing's syndrome. Steroid biosynthesis inhibitors are the most effective of these and can be used regardless of the cause. Metyrapone and etomidate are particularly useful in obtaining fast remission of clinical symptoms in severely ill or psychotic patients, and the latter has the advantage that it can used parenterally in patients unable or too unwell to tolerate oral medication. Our preferred treatments are metyrapone or ketoconazole either as monotherapy or in combination. The advantage of ketoconazole is its anti-androgenic action, particularly in women complaining of hirsutism. Careful monitoring of treatment is important, especially as all agents have the potential for precipitating hypoadrenalism. Occasionally, in difficult-to-control disease, we may institute a block-and-replace regime, using dexamethasone as the replacement glucocorticoid so that we can still monitor the endogenous cortisol production.

Neuromodulatory drugs have less of a role to play. However, they may be useful adjunctive agents in some cases of Cushing's disease or Nelson's syndrome, although it is likely to be a case of trial-and-error discovery of which agent may be effective in individual cases. Octreotide is potentially effective treatment in somatostatin receptor-positive ectopic ACTH-producing tumors.

REFERENCES

1. LAMBERTS, S.W. *et al.* 1995. Transsphenoidal selective adenomectomy is the treatment of choice in patients with Cushing's disease: considerations concerning preoperative medical treatment and the long-term follow-up. J. Clin. Endocrinol. Metab. **80:** 3111–3113.
2. LIDDLE, G.W. *et al.* 1959. Clinical application of a new test of pituitary reserve. J. Clin. Endocrinol. Metab. **19:** 875–894.
3. NEWELL-PRICE, J. *et al.* 1998. The diagnosis and differential diagnosis of Cushing's syndrome and pseudo-Cushing's states. Endocr. Rev. **19:** 647–672.
4. CARBALLEIRA, A. *et al.* 1976. Dual sites of inhibition by metyrapone of human adrenal steroidogenesis: correlation of *in vivo* and *in vitro* studies. J. Clin. Endocrinol. Metab. **42:** 687–695.
5. TRAINER, P.J. & M. BESSER. 1994. Cushing's syndrome: therapy directed at the adrenal glands. Endocrinol. Metab. Clin. N. Amer. **23:** 571–584.
6. VERHELST, J.A. *et al.* 1991 Short and long-term responses to metyrapone in the medical management of 91 patients with Cushing's syndrome. Clin. Endocrinol. (Oxf.) **35:** 169–178.
7. THOREN, M. *et al.* 1985. Aminoglutethimide and metyrapone in the management of Cushing's syndrome. Acta Endocrinol. (Copenh.) **109:** 451–457.
8. CHILD, D.F. *et al.* 1976. Drug controlled of Cushing's syndrome: combined aminoglutethimide and metyrapone therapy. Acta Endocrinol. (Copenh.) **82:** 330–341.
9. NUSSEY, S.S. *et al.* 1988. The combined use of sodium valproate and metyrapone in the treatment of Cushing's syndrome. Clin. Endocrinol. (Oxf.) **28:** 373–380.
10. ORTH, D.N. 1978. Metyrapone is useful only as adjunctive therapy in Cushing's disease. Ann. Intern. Med. **89:** 128–130.
11. JEFFCOATE, W.J. *et al.* 1977. Metyrapone in long-term management of Cushing's disease. Br. Med. J. **2:** 215–217.
12. DICKSTEIN, G. *et al.* 1986. Primary therapy for Cushing's disease with metyrapone. JAMA **255:** 1167–1169.
13. DONCKIER, J. *et al.* 1986. Successful control of Cushing's disease in the elderly with long term metyrapone. Postgrad. Med. J. **62:** 727–730.

14. CONNELL, J.M. et al. 1985. Pregnancy complicated by Cushing's syndrome: potential hazard of metyrapone therapy: case report. Br. J. Obstet. Gynaecol. **92:** 1192–1195.
15. SANTEN, R.J. et al. 1983. Site of action of low dose ketoconazole on androgen biosynthesis in men. J. Clin. Endocrinol. Metab. **57:** 732–736.
16. PONT, A. et al. 1985. Ketoconazole-induced increase in estradiol-testosterone ratio: probable explanation for gynecomastia. Arch. Intern. Med. **145:** 1429–1431.
17. ENGELHARDT, D. et al. 1985. Ketoconazole blocks cortisol secretion in man by inhibition of adrenal 11 beta-hydroxylase. Klin. Wochenschr. **63:** 607–612.
18. ENGELHARDT, D. et al. 1991 The influence of ketoconazole on human adrenal steroidogenesis: incubation studies with tissue slices. Clin. Endocrinol. (Oxf.) **35:** 163–168.
19. STEEN, R.E. et al. 1991 In vivo and in vitro inhibition by ketoconazole of ACTH secretion from a human thymic carcinoid tumour. Acta Endocrinol. (Copenh.) **125:** 331–334.
20. MORTIMER, R.H. et al. 1991 Ketoconazole and plasma and urine steroid levels in Cushing's disease. Clin. Exp. Pharmacol.Physiol. **18:** 563–569.
21. SONINO, N. et al. 1991. Ketoconazole treatment in Cushing's syndrome: experience in 34 patients. Clin. Endocrinol. (Oxf.) **35:** 347–352.
22. TABARIN, A. et al. 1991. Use of ketoconazole in the treatment of Cushing's disease and ectopic ACTH syndrome. Clin. Endocrinol. (Oxf.) **34:** 63–69.
23. CHOU, S.C. & J.D. LIN. 2000. Long-term effects of ketoconazole in the treatment of residual or recurrent Cushing's disease. Endocr.J. **47:** 401–406.
24. AHMED, M. et al. 2000. ACTH-producing pituitary cancer: experience at the King Faisal Specialist Hospital & Research Centre. Pituitary **3:** 105–112.
25. RICKMAN, T. et al. 2001. Hypokalemia, metabolic alkalosis, and hypertension: Cushing's syndrome in a patient with metastatic prostate adenocarcinoma. Am. J. Kidney Dis. **37:** 838–846.
26. LEWIS, J.H. et al. 1984. Hepatic injury associated with ketoconazole therapy: analysis of 33 cases. Gastroenterology **86:** 503–513.
27. STRICKER, B.H. et al. 1986. Ketoconazole-associated hepatic injury: a clinicopathological study of 55 cases. J. Hepatol. **3:** 399–406.
28. DUARTE, P.A. et al. 1984. Fatal hepatitis associated with ketoconazole therapy. Arch. Intern. Med. **144:** 1069–1070.
29. Knight, T.E. et al. 1991. Ketoconazole-induced fulminant hepatitis necessitating liver transplantation. J. Am..Acad. Dermatol. **25:** 398–400.
30. LAKE-BAKAAR, G. et al. 1987. Hepatic reactions associated with ketoconazole in the United Kingdom. Br. Med. J. (Clin. Res. Ed.) **294:** 419–422.
31. MCCANCE, D.R. et al. 1987. Acute hypoadrenalism and hepatotoxicity after treatment with ketoconazole. Lancet **1:** 573.
32. TUCKER, W.S., JR. et al. 1985. Reversible adrenal insufficiency induced by ketoconazole. JAMA **253:** 2413–2414.
33. MIETTINEN, T.A. 1988. Cholesterol metabolism during ketoconazole treatment in man. J. Lipid Res. **29:** 43–51.
34. DEXTER, R.N. et al. 1967. Inhibition of adrenal corticosteroid synthesis by aminoglutethimide: studies of the mechanism of action. J. Clin. Endocrinol. Metab. **27:** 473–480.

35. CASH, R. et al. 1967. Aminoglutethimide (Elipten-Ciba) as an inhibitor of adrenal steroidogenesis: mechanism of action and therapeutic trial. J. Clin. Endocrinol. Metab. **27:** 1239–1248.
36. SHAW, M.A. et al. 1988. Aminoglutethimide and ketoconazole: historical perspectives and future prospects. J. Steroid Biochem. **31:** 137–146.
37. FISHMAN, L.M. et al. 1967. Effects of amino-glutethimide on adrenal function in man. J. Clin. Endocrinol. Metab. **27:** 481–490.
38. MISBIN, R.I. et al. 1976. Aminoglutethimide in the treatment of Cushing's syndrome. J. Clin. Pharmacol. **16:** 645–651.
39. ZACHMANN, M. et al. 1977. Effect of aminoglutethimide on urinary cortisol and cortisol metabolites in adolescents with Cushing's syndrome. Clin. Endocrinol. (Oxf.) **7:** 63–71.
40. YOUNG, R.B. et al. 1973. Complexing of DDT and o,p'-DDD with adrenal cytochrome P-450 hydroxylating systems. J. Steroid Biochem. **4:** 585–591.
41. BERGENSTAL, D.M. et al. 1960. Chemotherapy of adrenocortical cancer with O,p'DDD. Ann. Intern. Med. **53:** 672–682.
42. LUTON, J.P. et al. 1990. Clinical features of adrenocortical carcinoma, prognostic factors, and the effect of mitotane therapy. N. Engl. J. Med. **322:** 1195–1201.
43. SOUTHREN, A.L. et al. 1961. Effect of O,p'DDD in a patient with Cushing's Syndrome. J. Clin. Endocrinol. Metab. **21:** 201–208.
44. LUTON, J.P. et al. 1979. Treatment of Cushing's disease by O,p'DDD. Survey of 62 cases. N. Engl. J. Med. **300:** 459–464.
45. HAAK, H.R. et al. 1991. Prolonged bleeding time due to mitotane therapy. Eur. J. Cancer **27:** 638–641.
46. VAN SETERS, A.P. & A.J. MOOLENAAR. 1991. Mitotane increases the blood levels of hormone-binding proteins. Acta Endocrinol. (Copenh.) **124:** 526–533.
47. MAHER, V.M. et al. 1992. Possible mechanism and treatment of o,p'-DDD-induced hypercholesterolaemia. Q. J. Med. **84:** 671–679.
48. LEDINGHAM, I.M. & I. WATT. 1983. Influence of sedation on mortality in critically ill multiple trauma patients. Lancet **1:** 1270.
49. WEBER, M.M. et al. 1993. Different inhibitory effect of etomidate and ketoconazole on the human adrenal steroid biosynthesis. Clin. Invest. **71:** 933–938.
50. LAMBERTS, S.W. et al. 1987. Differential effects of the imidazole derivatives etomidate, ketoconazole and miconazole and of metyrapone on the secretion of cortisol and its precursors by human adrenocortical cells. J. Pharmacol. Exp. Ther. **240:** 259–264.
51. DE COSTER, R. et al. 1985. Effects of etomidate on cortisol biosynthesis in isolated guinea-pig adrenal cells: comparison with metyrapone. J. Endocrinol. Invest. **8:** 199–202.
52. ALLOLIO, B. et al. 1983. Long-term etomidate and adrenocortical suppression. Lancet **2:** 626.
53. ALLOLIO, B. et al. 1988. Nonhypnotic low-dose etomidate for rapid correction of hypercortisolaemia in Cushing's syndrome. Klin. Wochenschr. **66:** 361–364.
54. HERRMANN, B.L. et al. 2001. [Transsphenoidal hypophysectomy of a patient with an ACTH-producing pituitary adenoma and an "empty sella" after pretreatment with etomidate]. Dtsch. Med. Wochenschr. **126:** 232–234.

55. DRAKE, W.M. et al. 1998. Emergency and prolonged use of intravenous etomidate to control hypercortisolemia in a patient with Cushing's syndrome and peritonitis. J. Clin. Endocrinol. Metab. **83:** 3542–3544.
56. KRAKOFF, J. et al. 2001. Use of a parenteral propylene glycol-containing etomidate preparation for the long-term management of ectopic Cushing's syndrome. J. Clin. Endocrinol. Metab. **86:** 4104–4108.
57. KRIEGER, D.T. & M. LURIA. 1976. Effectiveness of cyproheptadine in decreasing plasma ACTH concentrations in Nelson's syndrome. J. Clin. Endocrinol. Metab. **43:** 1179–1182.
58. SUDA, T. et al. 1983. Effects of cyproheptadine, reserpine, and synthetic corticotropin-releasing factor on pituitary glands from patients with Cushing's disease. J. Clin. Endocrinol. Metab. **56:** 1094–1099.
59. WAVEREN HOGERVORST, C.O. et al. 1996. Cortisol secretory patterns in Cushing's disease and response to cyproheptadine treatment. J. Clin. Endocrinol. Metab. **81:** 652–655.
60. TANAKOL, R. et al. 1996. Cyproheptadine treatment in Cushing's disease. J. Endocrinol. Invest. **19:** 242–247.
61. WHITEHEAD, H.M. et al. 1990. The effect of cyproheptadine and/or bromocriptine on plasma ACTH levels in patients cured of Cushing's disease by bilateral adrenalectomy. Clin. Endocrinol. (Oxf.) **32** : 193–201.
62. SONINO, N. et al. 1992. Potential therapeutic effects of ritanserin in Cushing's disease. JAMA **267:** 1073.
63. SONINO, N. et al. 2000. Effect of the serotonin antagonists ritanserin and ketanserin in Cushing's disease. Pituitary **3:** 55–59.
64. LAMBERTS, S.W. et al. 1980. The mechanism of the suppressive action of bromocriptine on adrenocorticotropin secretion in patients with Cushing's disease and Nelson's syndrome. J. Clin. Endocrinol. Metab. **51:** 307–311.
65. BOSCARO, M. et al. 1983. Effect of bromocriptine in pituitary-dependent Cushing's syndrome. Clin. Endocrino.l (Oxf.) **19:** 485–491.
66. MERCADO-ASIS, L.B. et al. 1992. Beneficial effects of high daily dose bromocriptine treatment in Cushing's disease. Endocrinol. Jpn. **39:** 385–395.
67. PIVONELLO, R. et al. 1999. Complete remission of Nelson's syndrome after 1-year treatment with cabergoline. J .Endocrinol. Invest. **22:** 860–865.
68. LAMBERTS, S.W. et al. 1982. Adrenocorticotropin-secreting pituitary adenomas originate from the anterior or the intermediate lobe in Cushing's disease: differences in the regulation of hormone secretion. J. Clin. Endocrinol. Metab. **54:** 286–291.
69. CROUGHS, R.J. et al. 1989. Bromocriptine-responsive Cushing's disease associated with anterior pituitary corticotroph hyperplasia or normal pituitary gland. J. Clin. Endocrinol. Metab. **68:** 495–498.
70. DE HERDER, W.W. & S.W. LAMBERTS. 1996. Is there a role for somatostatin and its analogs in Cushing's syndrome? Metabolism **45:** 83–85.
71. GREENMAN, Y. & S. MELMED. 1994. Heterogeneous expression of two somatostatin receptor subtypes in pituitary tumors. J. Clin. Endocrinol. Metab. **78:** 398–403.
72. LAMBERTS, S.W. et al. 1989 The effect of the long-acting somatostatin analogue SMS 201-995 on ACTH secretion in Nelson's syndrome and Cushing's disease. Acta Endocrinol. (Copenh.) **120:** 760–766.

73. BERTAGNA, X. *et al.* 1989. Suppression of ectopic adrenocorticotropin secretion by the long-acting somatostatin analog octreotide. J. Clin. Endocrinol. Metab. **68:** 988–991.
74. VIGNATI, F. & P. LOLI. 1996. Additive effect of ketoconazole and octreotide in the treatment of severe adrenocorticotropin-dependent hypercortisolism. J. Clin. Endocrinol. Metab. **81:** 2885–2890.
75. KOPPESCHAAr, H.P. *et al.* 1983. Sodium valproate and cyproheptadine may independently induce a remission in the same patient with Cushing's disease. Acta Endocrinol. (Copenh.) **104:** 160–163.
76. BECKERS, A. *et al.* 1990. Cyclical Cushing's disease and its successful control under sodium valproate. J. Endocrinol. Invest. **13:** 923–929.
77. GOMI, M. *et al.* 1985. Unaltered stimulation of pituitary adrenocorticotrophin secretion by corticotrophin-releasing factor following sodium valproate administration in a patient with Nelson's syndrome. Clin. Endocrinol. (Oxf.) **23:** 123–127.
78. COLAO, A. *et al.* 1997. Failure of long-term therapy with sodium valproate in Cushing's disease. J. Endocrinol. Invest. **20:** 387–392.
79. BAULIEU, E.E. 1991 The steroid hormone antagonist RU486. Mechanism at the cellular level and clinical applications. Endocrinol. Metab. Clin. N. Amer. **20:** 873–891.
80. HEALY, D.L. *et al.* 1985. Increased adrenocorticotropin, cortisol, and arginine vasopressin secretion in primates after the antiglucocorticoid steroid RU 486: dose response relationships. J. Clin. Endocrinol. Metab. **60:** 1–4.
81. BERTAGNA, X. *et al.* 1984. The new steroid analog RU 486 inhibits glucocorticoid action in man. J. Clin. Endocrinol. Metab. **59:** 25–28.
82. NIEMAN, L.K. *et al.* 1985. Successful treatment of Cushing's syndrome with the glucocorticoid antagonist RU 486. J. Clin. Endocrinol. Metab. **61:** 536–540.
83. BERTAGNA, X. *et al.* 1986. Pituitary-adrenal response to the antiglucocorticoid action of RU 486 in Cushing's syndrome. J. Clin. Endocrinol. Metab. **63:** 639–643.
84. SARTOR, O. & G.B.CUTLER, JR. 1996 Mifepristone: treatment of Cushing's syndrome. Clin. Obstet. Gynecol. **39:** 506–510.
85. TRAINER, P.J. *et al.* 1993. The relationship between cortisol production rate and serial serum cortisol estimation in patients on medical therapy for Cushing's syndrome. Clin. Endocrinol. (Oxf.) **39:** 441–443.
86. LACROIX, A. *et al.* 1992 Gastric inhibitory polypeptide-dependent cortisol hypersecretion: a new cause of Cushing's syndrome. N. Engl. J. Med. **327:** 974–980.
87. LACROIX, A. *et al.* 2000 The diversity of abnormal hormone receptors in adrenal Cushing's syndrome allows novel pharmacological therapies. Braz. J.Med. Biol. Res. **33:** 1201–1209.
88. PAEZ-PEREDA, M. *et al.* 2001 Retinoic acid prevents experimental Cushing syndrome. J. Clin. Invest. **108:** 1123–1131.

Association of Hypertension and Hypokalemia with Cushing's Syndrome Caused by Ectopic ACTH Secretion

A Series of 58 Cases

DAVID J. TORPY,[a] NANCY MULLEN,[b] IOANNIS ILIAS,[c] AND LYNNETTE K. NIEMAN[c]

[a]*University of Queensland, Department of Medicine, Greenslopes Hospital, Brisbane, Queensland 4120, Australia*

[b]*Department of Nursing, Clinical Center, National Institutes of Health, Bethesda, Maryland 20892, USA*

[c]*Pediatric and Reproductive Endocrinology Branch, National Institutes of Child Health and Human Development, National Institutes of Health, Bethesda, Maryland 20892-1583, USA*

> ABSTRACT: Cushing's syndrome is associated with hypertension in approximately 80% of cases. Hypertension contributes to the marked increased mortality risk of past or current Cushing's syndrome, largely because of increased cardiovascular risk. Observation of the pathophysiological effect of chronically elevated ACTH and cortisol values in patients with ectopic ACTH secretion complements the available data from acute studies of the effects of ACTH and glucocorticoid infusions in normal volunteers. In a retrospective case review, we identified 58 patients with Cushing's syndrome caused by ectopic ACTH secretion, who were treated at the National Institutes of Health between 1983–1997. The diagnosis of an ectopic ACTH cause was confirmed by inferior petrosal sinus sampling and/or pathologic examination of tumor. The commonest causes were bronchial carcinoid (40%) and thymic carcinoid (10%), but 18 of 58 (31%) patients had an unknown source of ectopic ACTH. Hypertension (systolic blood pressure >140 mmHg and/or diastolic blood pressure >90 mmHg in adults) was noted in 45 of 58 (78%) ectopic Cushing's patients, a prevalence similar to that noted in other endogenous Cushing's syndrome etiologies. Hypertension was severe, deemed to require 3 or more drugs by the treating physicians, in 26 of 58 (45%) patients. Hypokalemia was much more prevalent than in patients with other causes of Cushing's syndrome, affecting 33 of 58 (57%) patients. The range of plasma ACTH

Address for correspondence: David J. Torpy, University of Queensland Department of Medicine, Greenslopes Hospital, Newdegate Street, Brisbane, Qld. 4120, Australia
dtorpy@mailbox.uq.edu.au

(17–1557 pg/mL, normal <60) and 24-hour urine cortisol (UC) excretion (192–1600 mcg/24 hr, normal <90) allowed analysis of the influence of these hormones on blood pressure and plasma potassium. There was a significant relationship between 24-hour UC excretion and the presence of hypokalemia ($P = 0.003$). Eight of nine patients with a UC >6000 mcg/24 hr had hypokalemia. There was no relation between ACTH level and hypokalemia. In addition, we did not find blood pressure severity to be related to UC excretion or ACTH levels. Urine and plasma cortisol and cortisol metabolite measurements suggest that cortisol may act as a mineralocorticoid when in excess, perhaps by saturating the 11β-hydroxysteroid-dehydrogenase (11β-HSD2 enzyme) that inactivates cortisol at the renal tubule. The current data suggest that high cortisol levels may be the principal cause of hypokalemic alkalosis in Cushing's syndrome, rather than inhibition of the 11βHSD2 enzyme by ACTH or the effects of adrenal steroid biosynthetic intermediaries with mineralococorticoid activity.

KEYWORDS: corticotropin; hypertension; hypokalemia; 11β-hydroxysteroid-dehydrogenase

INTRODUCTION

Cushing's syndrome due to autonomous ACTH secretion from an extrapituitary source, first described in 1965, causes 5–10% of cases of spontaneous Cushing's syndrome.[1,2] Hypertension is a frequent feature of Cushing's syndrome, occurring in 80% of all cases. In addition, severe hypercortisolism is associated with hypokalemic alkalosis. We conducted a retrospective case review of patients with Cushing's syndrome caused by ectopic ACTH secretion. As these patients have a spectrum of hypercortisolism, our intent was to correlate the severity of hypercortisolism with the severity of hypertension and hypokalemia.

METHODS

A retrospective case review identified 58 patients (24 male, 34 female; mean age ± SD: 36 ± 17 years old; age range: 10–69 years) with ectopic ACTH secretion diagnosed and treated at the Warren Grant Magnuson Clinical Center at the National Institutes of Health. Fifty patients were Caucasians, five were Hispanics and three were African-Americans. Mean BMI ± SD was 30.0 ± 8.0 kg/m^2. All patients had ACTH-dependent hypercortisolism as indicated by elevated urine cortisol (UC) excretion, and normal to elevated plasma ACTH concentration. Inferior petrosal sinus sampling was performed in most patients (45 of 58; 78%) and excluded a pituitary ACTH source. Other cases were confirmed by resection of likely ACTH-secreting

TABLE 1. Final diagnosis of ACTH source based on surgical biopsy or excision in 58 consecutive causes of Cushing's syndrome due to ectopic ACTH secretion

Diagnosis	Patients (total = 58)
Bronchial carcinoid	23 (40%)
Carcinoid tumorlets	1 (2%)
Thymic carcinoid	6 (10%)
Metastatic gastrinoma	3 (5%)
Pheochromocytoma	2 (3%)
Medullary thyroid carcinoma	2 (4%)
Neuroendocinre tumor of the carotid sheath	1 (2%)
Islet cell neuroendocrine tumor	1 (2%)
Small cell carcinoma of the lung	1 (2%)
Unknown	18 (31%)

tumor. Localization of the ACTH source was based on imaging (computed tomography, magnetic resonance imaging, octreotide scintigraphy, and/or ultrasound) and invasive investigations (e.g., arteriography, venous sampling) followed by surgical excision or biopsy. The influence of octreotide scintigraphy on diagnosis in a subset of this patient group is described elsewhere.[3]

The source of ACTH as confirmed by pathologic examination of tumor is summarized in TABLE 1. The series had relatively few cases of frank malignant sources of ACTH, reflecting study entry criteria. In addition, the number of cases with an unknown ACTH source was higher than other smaller series (18 of 58; 31%), probably reflecting referral bias towards the more difficult case.[4,5] The commonest causes were bronchial carcinoid (23 of 58; 40%) and thymic carcinoid (6 of 58; 10%).

Blood pressure (BP) was assessed from inpatient automated oscillometric recordings (Dinamap, Critikon, Tampa, FL) generally taken 2–4 times daily. Plasma ACTH and UC levels were measured by conventional radioimmunoassay and immunoflourometric assay, as previously described.[6] Most patients were admitted to the Clinical Center for at least 2 weeks. In adults, systolic BP persistently over 140 mmHg and/or diastolic BP persistently over 90 mmHg was regarded as hypertension, while in children hypertension was diagnosed on the basis of available age-based nomograms. Hypertension was classified as mild to moderate if patients were taking one or two anti-hypertensive drugs and severe if three or more anti-hypertensives were deemed necessary by the treating physician. Hypokalemia was defined as plasma potassium < 3.5 mmol/L. Most patients had been treated with sufficient potassium supplements to increase plasma potassium to the normal range. Data between groups of Cushing's patients was compared using analysis of vari-

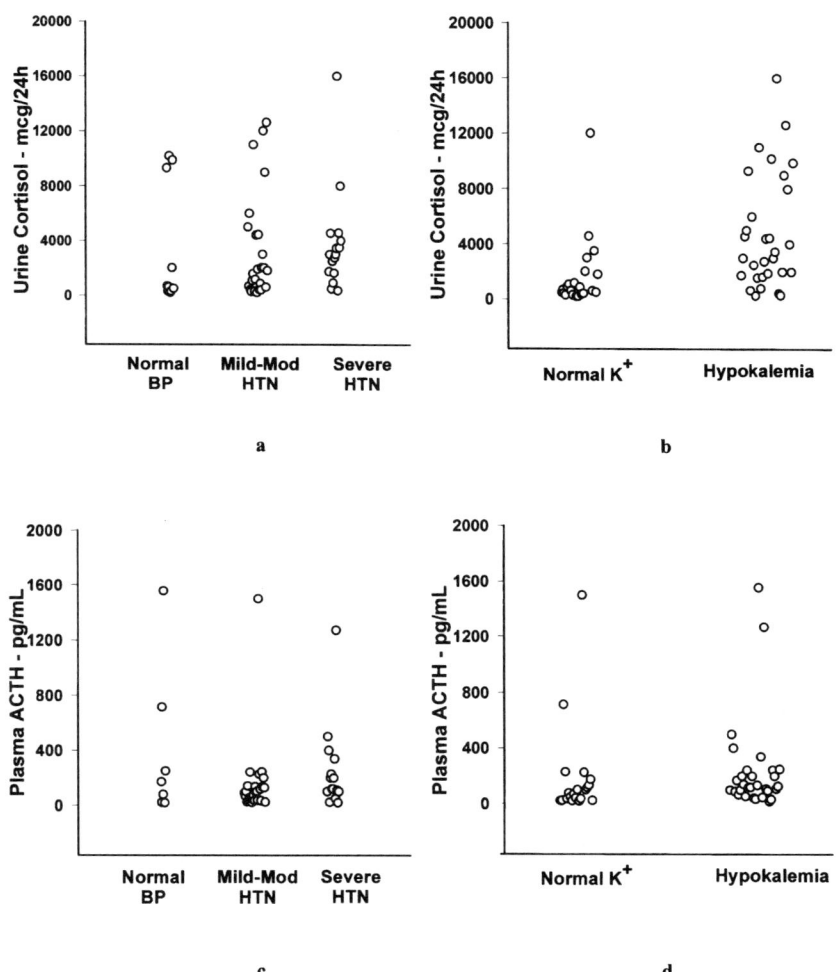

FIGURE 1. (**a**) Urine cortisol levels (normal range < 90 mcg/24 hr) in Cushing's patients with normal blood pressure (BP, $n = 10$), mild to moderate (Mild-Mod) hypertension (HTN) requiring 1–2 antihypertensives ($n = 28$) and patients with severe hypertension ($n = 17$). There did not appear to be a close relationship between cortisol excretion rates and hypertension severity. (**b**) Urine cortisol levels in normokalemic ($n = 21$) and hypokalemic ($n = 30$) cases of Cushing's syndrome due to ectopic ACTH secretion. There was a significant difference in urine cortisol between hypokalemic and normokalemic cases (4749 ± 754 vs. 1633 ± 553 mcg/24 hr, $P = 0.003$). (**c**) ACTH levels related to hypertension severity. Plasma ACTH levels as shown in normotensive ($n = 7$), mild to moderate hypertensive ($n = 26$), and severely hypertensive ($n = 17$) subjects with Cushing's syndrome due to ectopic ACTH secretion. (**d**) ACTH levels in normokalemic ($n = 21$) and hypokalemic ($n = 30$) subjects with Cushing's syndrome due to ectopic ACTH secretion.

ance (ANOVA), independent *t* tests and the Chi square test, while correlations were analyzed by Spearman's rank correlation.

RESULTS

Hypertension was present in 45 of 58 (78%) patients. Hypertension was mild to moderate in 26 of 58 (45%) patients and severe in 19 of 58 (33%) patients. Three patients had hypertension prior to the development of other clinical features of hypercortisolism; two of these had severe hypertension.

There was a wide range of severity of hypercortisolism (UC: 192–16,000 mcg/24 hr, reference range < 90, mean ± SE: 3430 ± 502 mcg/24 hr). Plasma ACTH values also ranged widely (17–1557 pg/ml, mean ± SE: 187 ± 37 pg/ml, reference range < 60 pg/ml). There was no significant correlation between plasma ACTH and UC levels (r: +0.20, $P > 0.10$). Urine cortisol levels did not correlate with hypertension severity (FIG. 1a; $P > 0.10$, ANOVA). However, cortisol excretion rates did relate to the presence or absence of hypokalemia (FIG. 1b), since UC levels were significantly higher in hypokalemic than in normokalemic patients (mean ± SE: 4749 ± 754 vs. 1633 ± 553 mcg/24 hr, $P = 0.003$, ANOVA). Extremely high UC levels (>4000 mcg/24 hr) were generally associated with hypokalemia. In contrast, plasma ACTH levels did not appear to relate to the severity of hypertension (FIG. 1c) or the presence of hypokalemia (FIG. 1d; both $P > 0.10$, ANOVA).

There was no relation between age and the presence of mild or severe hypertension or between BMI and hypertension (all $P > 0.10$, ANOVA).

Impaired glucose (IGT) tolerance or diabetes mellitus (DM) of recent onset accompanied Cushing's syndrome symptoms in 22 of 58 patients, while a single patient had a history of long-standing DM. However, IGT or DM were not related to HT (odds ratio: 1.64, $P = 0.45$; Chi square).

DISCUSSION

Our data suggest that the severity of hypercortisolism in ectopic ACTH syndrome influences the frequency of hypokalemia but not hypertension. Hypokalemia was frequent in our series, at 57%, compared to approximately 10% in pituitary-dependent Cushing's syndrome.[5] Hypokalemia was almost universal at very high UC levels (>40 times normal) and UC levels were significantly higher in the hypokalemic group compared to normokalemic subjects.

The cause(s) of hypokalemia in Cushing's syndrome are not fully understood. Cortisol can act as a mineralocorticoid, as its *in vitro* binding affinity to the mineralocorticoid receptor is equal to that of aldosterone.[7] Cortisol circulates in blood at a 1000-fold concentration greater than aldosterone, but is approximately 95% bound to its own specific binding globulin (corticosteroid binding globulin). The mineralocorticoid receptor in the renal tubule is protected from this apparent excess of cortisol by the action of 11β-hydroxysteroid-dehydrogenase (11β-HSD2) to convert cortisol to inactive cortisone.[7] A congenital deficiency of 11β-HSD2, described in approximately 50 cases worldwide, explains the condition of apparent mineralocorticoid excess where plasma renin activity and aldosterone are suppressed.[9] Inhibition of the enzyme by liquorice (glycyrrhizic acid) or carbenoxolone also can produce a reversible mineralocorticoid excess state.[10]

Thus, the mineralocorticoid excess-like state of the ectopic ACTH syndrome may be caused by supraphysiologic cortisol levels. These high cortisol levels may saturate the cortisol-inactivating enzyme, 11β-HSD2, at the renal tubule thereby allowing access of intact cortisol to the renal tubular mineralocorticoid receptor.[11]

ACTH has been thought to contribute directly to the mineralocorticoid excess-like state of ACTH-dependent Cushing's syndrome. ACTH may inhibit 11β-HSD2 either directly or by stimulating an inhibitory adrenal product.[12,13] Finally, it has been suggested that elevated corticosterone and deoxycorticosteroid (DOC), which possess mineralocorticoid activity, may correlate with hypokalemia in Cushing's syndrome.[14]

There is some *in vivo* evidence of an inhibitory effect of ACTH, or an ACTH product other than cortisol, on 11β-HSD2. Infusions of cortisol or ACTH in doses sufficient to produce Cushing's-like elevations of plasma cortisol in healthy volunteers have different effects on plasma cortisone levels. Cortisone levels rose with cortisol infusion, but rose less with ACTH infusion.[12] However, as ACTH does not directly inhibit 11β-HSD2 *in vitro*, the *in vivo* effect may be due to an adrenal product, such as cortisol.

Arguing against a major hypokalemic role for DOC and corticosterone are the observations that both hormones are elevated in normokalemic patients with Cushing's disease.[15] Although DOC levels in Cushing's syndrome are slightly elevated, they do not reach the levels seen in DOC-secreting tumors or the two forms of congenital adrenal hyperplasia, 11β-hydroxylase deficiency and 17α-hydroxylase deficiency. Therefore, DOC levels are probably too low to contribute greatly to the mineralocorticoid excess-like state seen with ectopic ACTH secretion.[12] The activity of 11β-HSD2 can be inferred by the ratio of cortisol metabolites tetrahydrocortisol (THF) + 5α-THF to tetrahydroxortisone (THE) in urine. This ratio is elevated in Cushing's syndrome patients, especially if they are hypokalemic.[16] The ratio of (THF + 5α-THF): THE correlates with both hypokalemia and elevated erythrocyte Na^+-H^+ exchange, a measure of functional mineralocorticoid excess.[17] A study of ectopic ($n = 9$) and non-ectopic ($n = 13$) ACTH-dependent Cushing's syndrome patients revealed an elevated ratio of (THF + 5α-THF): THE in ectopic compared to eutopic ACTH patients, although there was some overlap.[18]

Plasma potassium correlated significantly with UC and (THF + THF): THE ratio.

The plasma cortisol-to-cortisone ratio also may be used to infer peripheral 11β-HSD2 activity, particularly as selective venous sampling in volunteers has shown that the kidney is the principal source of cortisone.[12] In one study, nine ectopic ACTH syndrome patients had much higher plasma cortisol:cortisone ratios than did other Cushing's syndrome patients. This suggests inhibition of renal 11β-HSD2, either by cortisol saturation, or ACTH. Such a mechanism would explain the positive relationship between the elevated cortisol and hypokalemia in our patients.

In contrast to the relationship between cortisol and hypokalemia we found no correlation between urinary cortisol and hypertension. Stewart and colleagues also failed to find a relationship between urine cortisol or plasma cortisol:cortisone ratio and the extent of hypertension.[18] Those workers directly examined the association between cortisol levels and hypertension, although 23% of the patients were taking hypertensives, which the authors believe may have obscured any association. In our study, most patients were taking antihypertensives, so we examined the UC levels relative to number of antihypertensives employed and found no association. One limitation of our approach is that it does not take into account the likelihood of varying efficacy of different drug classes between patients and the possibility that patients' physicians may have slightly different goals for BP control.

In keeping with a lack of correlation between BP and adrenal products, our data suggest that the prevalence of hypertension among hypercortisolemic patients with ectopic ACTH secretion (78%) is similar to that in other series of Cushing's syndrome with other etiologic bases.[2] Early studies suggesting that hypertension was less prevalent in ectopic ACTH secretion may have been confounded by a preponderance of malignant cases, with attendant hypotension of disseminated malignancy.[14]

A study of 70 Cushing's syndrome patients found that the presence of hypertension has high discriminative value in separating Cushing's syndrome on clinical grounds from simple obesity. The value of hypertension was considered to be exceeded only by bruising and myopathy, although these features are usually seen much later in the course of Cushing's syndrome as they represent catabolic effects of longer-term excess glucocorticoid exposure.[19]

Hypertension is strongly associated with overall Cushing's syndrome mortality, unrelated to an ectopic ACTH etiology. An epidemiologic study in the region of Vizcaya, Spain that identified 49 patients diagnosed with Cushing's disease (1975–1992), 87.5% of whom achieved remission, revealed an overall mortality risk of 3.8 times the population average. This excess mortality is thought to be mainly due to an increased cardiovascular disease risk five times the population average.[20] A similar excess mortality was observed in a Danish population study of Cushing's syndrome, with a standardized mortality rate of 3.68, but this excess mortality was observed mainly during the first year of disease.[21]

In general, hypertension has been thought to be difficult to treat in the setting of Cushing's syndrome without direct relief from hypercortisolism. Blood pressure normalization was achieved in only four of 28 patients using calcium channel blockers, diuretic agents, or angiotensin-converting enzyme inhibitors.[22] However, hypertension generally responds well to ketoconazole, which lowers cortisol levels, RU486, which acts as an antagonist to the glucocorticoid receptor, or surgical cure.[22,23] Preoperative BP and duration of hypertension predict postoperative BP.[24,25]

Hypertension becomes more common with advancing age. While no relationship between age and presence of hypertension was noted in our patients, the patients we studied had a mean age of only 36 years. Obesity is associated with hypertension and may be a measure of the chronicity of patients' hypercortisolism. However, although the mean body mass index (BMI) of patients was in the obese range, a substantial number of them were not obese; hence we can understand the lack of relationship between BMI and hypertension.

Hypertension is common among diabetics. The same pathogenetic mechanisms are considered to apply in patients with DM, as well as in subjects with insulin resistance, and the activated renin–angiotensin system is thought to contribute to high BP.[26] From our results, the lack of any relationship between IGT or DM and hypertension in patients with ectopic Cushing's points to hypercortisolism as the unique causal factor of high BP in these patients.

If cortisol does not directly account for hypertension in Cushing's syndrome, what might account for this abnormality? Blood pressure represents the interaction of plasma volume, vascular tone, and cardiac output. Cardiac output and peripheral resistance are increased in Cushing's syndrome, but total exchangeable sodium is normal.[15] Ambulatory BP measures show a reduced nocturnal fall in Cushing's syndrome.[27] Cushing's syndrome patients tend to have suppressed levels of atrial natriuretic peptide (ANP), suggesting the presence of increased plasma sodium and volume. Angiotensinogen (renin substrate) levels, however, are approximately twice normal in Cushing's syndrome, due to a direct effect of glucocorticoids on the liver, although these should not ultimately influence functional mineralocorticoid status.[28,29] While acute ACTH administration transiently stimulates aldosterone secretion, in Cushing's syndrome both aldosterone and plasma renin activities are normal to low, suggesting that the aldosterone/renin system is not the cause of the mineralocorticoid type of hypertension which may be seen.

Glucocorticoids have an important permissive effect on vascular tone through several mechanisms. Increased pressor responses to noradrenaline and angiotensin II, and greater negative chronotropism with phenylephrine have been demonstrated in Cushing's syndrome patients.[29,30] Catecholamine concentrations in plasma and urine are normal in Cushing's syndrome.[15,31]

Glucocorticoids inhibit nitric oxide synthase, thereby reducing levels of nitric oxide, a well-known vasodilator.[32] Conversely, the hypotension and pressor non-responsive state seen in hypoadrenalism may be due to overproduction of nitric oxide.[33] The vasodilators PGE2 and kallikrein were reduced in patients with Cushing's syndrome.[29] Atrial natriuretic peptide also decreases vascular tone, and the effects of this appear to be relatively blocked in the presence of hypercortisolism.[34] Some vasoconstrictors which appear to be increased by glucocorticoids *in vitro* include vascular smooth muscle endothelin[35] and increased calcium influx to vessel walls.[36]

In summary, Cushing's syndrome caused by ectopic ACTH secretion is associated with similar rates of hypertension as those seen in other forms of endogenous hypercortisolism, but a state of functional mineralocorticoid excess may be more common. While the severity of hypercortisolism does not predict the severity of hypertension, our data and those of others show that hypokalemia correlates with cortisol levels. Studies of urine and plasma cortisol, cortisone, and their metabolites have inferred an inhibition of kidney 11β-HSD2 in patients with ectopic ACTH secretion, probably related to the degree of hypercortisolism, allowing cortisol to act as a mineralocorticoid. Saturation of kidney 11β-HSD2 by circulating glucocorticoid may allow cortisol to reach the mineralocorticoid receptor and produce the state of mineralocorticoid excess seen in these patients. The correlation of hypokalemia with cortisol levels within cases of ectopic Cushing's syndrome in larger series supports this explanation. While there is evidence of relative 11β-HSD2 inactivity, which may relate directly or indirectly to ACTH excess, hypercortisolism with subsequent 11β-HSD2 enzyme saturation seems to be the principal cause of functional mineralocorticoid excess in Cushing's syndrome.

REFERENCES

1. LIDDLE, G.W., GIVENS, J.R., NICHOLSON, W.E. & D.P. ISLAND. 1965. The ectopic ACTH syndrome. Cancer Res. **25:** 1057–1061.
2. NIEMAN, L.K. 1997. Cushing's syndrome. Curr. Ther. Endocrinol. Metab. **6:** 161–164.
3. TORPY, D.J., C.C. CHEN, N. MULLEN, *et al.* 1999. Lack of utility of 111-In-pentetreotide scintigraphy in localizing ectopic ACTH producing tumors: follow-up of 18 patients. J. Clin. Endocrinol. Metab. **84:** 1186–1192.
4. JEX, R.K., J.A. VAN HEERDEN, P.C. CARPENTER & C.S. GRANT. 1985. Ectopic ACTH syndrome: diagnostic and therapeutic aspects. Am. J. Surg. **149:** 276–282.
5. HOWLETT, T.A., P.L. DRURY, L. PERRY, *et al.* 1986. Diagnosis and management of ACTH dependent Cushing's syndrome: comparison of the features of ectopic and pituitary ACTH production. Clin. Endocrinol. (Oxf). **24:** 699–713.

6. PAPANICOLAOU, D.A., C. TSIGOS, E.H. OLDFIELD & G.P. CHROUSOS. 1996. Acute glucocorticoid deficiency is associated with plasma elevations of interleukin-6: does the latter participate in the symptomatology of the steroid withdrawal syndrome and adrenal insufficiency? J. Clin. Endocrinol. Metab. **81:** 2303–2306.
7. KROZOWSKI, Z.S. & J.W. FUNDER. 1983. Renal mineralocorticoid receptors and hippocampal corticosterone-binding species have identical intrinsic steroid specificity. Proc. Natl. Acad. Sci. USA **80:** 6065–6060.
8. FUNDER, J.W., P.T. PEARCE, R. SMITH & A.I. SMITH. 1988. Mineralocorticoid action: target tissue specificity is enzyme, not receptor, mediated. Science **242:** 583–585.
9. STEWART, P.M., J.E.T. CORRIE, C.H.L. SHACKLETON & C.R.W. EDWARDS. 1988. Syndrome of apparent mineralocorticoid excess: a defect in the cortisol: cortisone shuttle. J. Clin. Invest. **82:** 340–349.
10. STEWART, P.M., A.M. WALLACE, R. VALENTINO, et al. 1987. Mineralocorticoid activity of licorice: 11β-hydroxysteroid dehydrogenase deficiency comes of age. Lancet **2:** 821–824.
11. ULICK, S., J.Z. WANG, J.D. BLUMENFELD & T.G. PICKERING. 1992. Cortisol inactivation overload: a mechanism of mineralocorticoid hypertension in the ectopic adrenocorticotropin syndrome. J. Clin. Endocrinol. Metab. **74:** 963–967.
12. WALKER, B.R., J.C. CAMPBELL, R. FRASER, et al. 1992. Mineralocorticoid excess and inhibition of 11 beta-hydroxysteroid dehydrogenase in patients with ectopic ACTH syndrome. Clin. Endocrinol. (Oxf.). **37:** 481–482.
13. RUSVAI, A.N. & A.N. FEJES-TOTH. 1993. A new isoform of 11ß-hydroxysteroid dehydrogenase in aldosterone target cells. J. Biol. Chem. **268:** 10717–10720.
14. SCHAMBELAN, M., P.E. SLATON & E.G. BIGLIERI. 1971. Mineralocorticoid production in hyper-adrenocortisicism. Role in pathogenesis of hypokalemic alkalosis. Am. J. Med. **51:** 299–303.
15. RITCHIE, C.M., B. SHERIDAN, R. FRASER, et al. 1990. Studies on the pathogenesis of hypertension in Cushing's disease and acromegaly. Q. J. Med. **280:** 855–867.
16. HERMUS, A., S. HOBMA, G. PIETERS, et al. 1991. Are the hypokalaemia and hypertension in Cushing's disease caused by apparent mineralocorticoid excess? Horm. Metab. Res. **23:** 572–573.
17. KOREN, W., A. GRIENSPUHN, S.R. KUZNETSOV, et al. 1998. Enhanced Na^+/H^+ exchange in Cushing's syndrome reflects functional hypermineralocorticoidism. J. Hypertens. **16:** 1187–1191.
18. STEWART, P.M., V.R. WALKER, G. HOLDER, et al. 1995. 11 beta-hydroxysteroid dehydrogenase activity in Cushing's syndrome: explaining the mineralocorticoid excess state of the ectopic adrenocorticotropin syndrome. J. Clin. Endocrinol. Metab. **80:** 3617–3620.
19. ROSS, E.J. & D.C. LINCH. 1982. Cushing's syndrome—killing disease: discrimination value of signs and symptoms aiding early diagnosis. Lancet **2:** 646–649.
20. ETXABE, J. & J.A. VAZQUEZ. 1994. Morbidity and mortality in Cushing's disease: an epidemiological approach. Clin. Endocrinol. (Oxf.). **40:** 479–484.

21. LINDHOLM, J., S. JUUL, J.O. JORGENSEN, et al. 2001. Incidence and late prognosis of Cushing's syndrome: a population-based study. J. Clin. Endocrinol. Metab. **86:** 117–123.
22. FALLO, F., A. PAOLETTA, F. TONA, et al. 1993. Response of hypertension to conventional antihypertensive treatment and/or steroidogenesis inhibitors in Cushing's syndrome. J. Intern. Med. **234:** 595–598.
23. LUDECKE, D.K. & G. NIEDWOROK. 1985. Results of microsurgery in Cushing's disease and effect on hypertension. Cardiology 72 (Suppl.1): 91–94.
24. FALLO, F., N. SONINO, L. BARZON, et al. 1996. Effect of surgical treatment on hypertension in Cushing's syndrome. Am. J. Hypertens. **9:** 77–80.
25. SUZUKI, T., H. SHIBATA, T. ANDO, et al. 2000. Risk factors associated with persistent post-operative hypertension in Cushing's syndrome. Endocr. Res. **26:** 791–795.
26. KIRPICHNIKOV, D. & J.R. SOWERS. 2001. Diabetes mellitus and diabetes-associated vascular disease. Trends Endocrinol. Metab. **12:** 225–230.
27. PADFIELD, P.L. & M.J. STEWART. 1991. Ambulatory blood pressure monitoring in secondary hypertension. J. Hypertens. **9** (Suppl 8): S69–S71.
28. REID, I.A. 1977. Effect of angiotensin II and glucocorticoids on plasma angiotensinogen concentration in the dog. Am. J. Physiol. **232:** E234–236.
29. SARUTA, T., H. SUZUKI, M. HANDA, et al. 1986. Multiple factors contribute to the pathogenesis of hypertension in Cushing's syndrome. J. Clin. Endocrinol. Metab. **62:** 275–279.
30. MCKNIGHT, J.A., D.P. ROONEY, H. WHITEHEAD & A.B. ATKINSON. 1995. Blood pressure responses to phenylephrine infusions in subjects with Cushing's syndrome. J. Hum. Hypertens. **9:** 855–858.
31. TENSHERT, W., P. BAUMGART, P. GREMINGER, et al. 1985. Pathogenetic aspects of hypertension in Cushing's syndrome. Cardiology **72** (Suppl 1): 84–90.
32. RADOMSKI, M.W., R.M.J. PALMER & S. MONCADA. 1990. Glucocorticoids inhibit the expression of inducible, but not the constitutive, nitric oxide synthase in vascular endothelial cells. Proc. Natl. Acad. Sci. USA **87:** 10043–10047.
33. ORBACH, P., C.E. WOOD & M. KELLER-WOOD. 2001. Nitric oxide reduces pressor responsiveness during ovine hypoadrenocorticism. Clin. Exp. Pharmacol. Physiol. **28:** 459–462.
34. YASUNARI, K., M. KOHNO, K. MURAKAWA, et al. 1990. Glucocorticoids and atrial natriuretic factor receptors on vascular smooth muscle. Hypertension **16:** 581–586.
35. KANSE, S.M., K. TAKAHASHI, J.B. WARREN, et al.. 1991. Glucocrticoids induce endothelin release from vascular smooth muscle cells but not endothelial cells. Eur. J. Pharmacol. **199:** 99–101.
36. HAYASHI, T., NAKAI, T. & S. MIYABO. 1991. Glucocorticoids increase Ca^{2+} uptake and [^{3}H]dihydropyridine binding in A7r5 vascular smooth muscle cells. Am. J. Physiol. **261**(1 Pt 1): C106–C114.

Hypertension in Congenital Adrenal Hyperplasia and Apparent Mineralocorticoid Excess

MARIA I. NEW

*Department of Pediatrics, Weill Cornell Medical College,
New York Presbyterian Hospital, Nwe York, New York 10021, USA*

ABSTRACT: Most often, low-renin hypertension in the child or adolescent has a clearly definable hormonal cause; thus while each of its numerous forms is moderately rare, a specific hormonal basis is to be expected. An endocrine evaluation is indicated after exclusion of cardiologic pathology or renovascular or portal abnormality in a hypertensive child. The evaluation should include analysis of catecholamine and of thyroid hormone plasma levels, and plasma renin activity (PRA) level. Hormonal hypertension with high or normal renin conditions is rare. Elevated blood pressure with high or normal renin levels may be in fact within normal range in the context of growth at upper percentile limits, possibly in conjunction with simple obesity. Diagnosis may be made at any age in most forms of low-renin hypertension.

KEYWORDS: congenital adrenal hyperplasia; CYP11B2; apparent mineralocorticoid excess; hypertension; low-renin hypertension; HSD11B2; children

Two carefully studied diseases causing childhood hypertension with suppressed renin are congenital adrenal hyperplasia (CAH) owing to 11β–hydroxylase deficiency and apparent mineralocorticoid excess (AME; TABLE 1). CAH and AME have a well-defined genetic basis and the loci concerned are autosomal, and thus both sexes are affected equally. In contrast to the rarity with which these disorders are found, their pathologic mechanisms may

---

Address for correspondence: Maria I. New, M.D., Department of Pediatrics, Weill Cornell Medical College, New York Presbyterian Hospital, 525 E. 68th Street, M622, New York, NY 10021. Voice: 212-746-3450; fax: 212-746-0300
   minew@med.cornell.edu

TABLE 1. Forms of endocrine hypertension with suppressed renin

Disorder	Signs and Symptoms	Hormonal Findings	Source	Genetics
Steroid 11β-hydroxylase deficiency	Ambiguous external genitalia in newborn females; precocious isosexual development/virilization, and accelerated growth in both sexes	Decreased PRA and aldosterone; elevated serum androgens/urine 17-ketosteroids; elevated DOC and 11-deoxycortisol (S)	Glandular: ZF of adrenal cortex	Mutations in gene CYP11B1 (which encodes cytochrome P450$_{11\beta/18}$ of ZF) impair synthesis of cortisol and ZF 17-deoxysteroids
Apparent mineralocorticoid excess (AME)	Cardiac conduction changes; +LVH and vessel remodeling. Some Ca ion abnormalities: nephrocalcinosis	Low plasma ACTH and secretory rates of all corticosteroids; serum F normal because of delayed plasma clearance. Extreme hypokalemia and severe hypertension aggravated by any sodium intake—or by hydrocortisone or ACTH—and responding to spironolactone	High F bioreactivity in periphery due to defective conversion of F→E owing to defective 11β-hydroxy-steroid dehydrogenase type 2 activity	Mutations in the gene, 11$BHSD2$, encoding enzyme 11β-hydroxy-steroid dehydrogenase 2

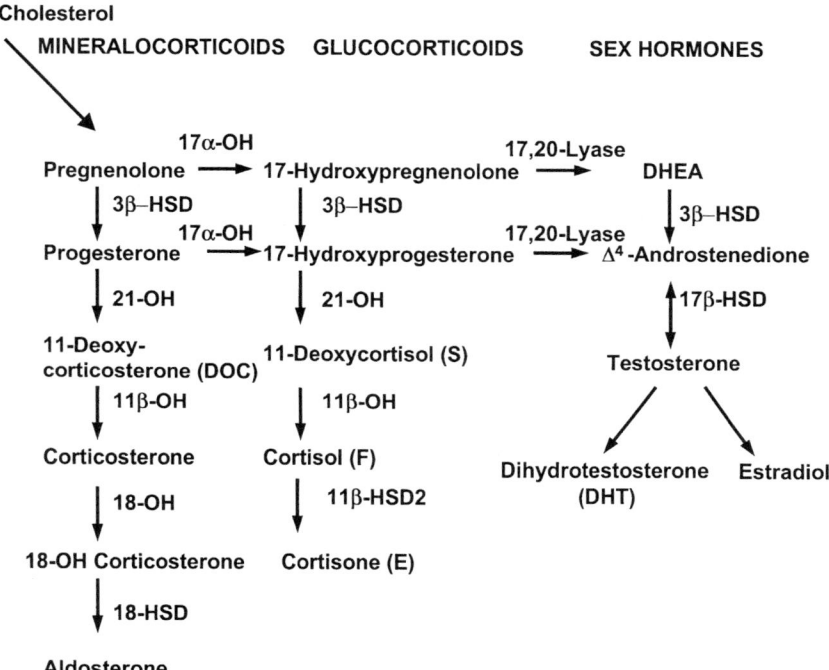

FIGURE 1. Simplified schema for adrenal steroidogenesis. (From New and White.[36] Reprinted by permission.)

prove to be operative to a mild degree in cases of essential hypertension in adult age, for which the genetic bases are currently being studied.[1]

STEROID 11β-HYDROXYLASE DEFICIENCY

An adrenal defect in any of the cortisol biosynthetic enzymes, because of the feedback relationship between the pituitary and adrenal, will induce a secondary increase in plasma ACTH that then drives the zona fasciculata (ZF) to produce cortisol precursors and other steroids in excess, according to the position of the enzymatic block in the adrenal steroidogenic scheme (FIG. 1). These enzymatic defects as a group are termed congenital adrenal hyperplasia (CAH). Each form of CAH specifically produces a characteristic plasma and excreted steroid profile and clinical picture.[2,3] The adrenal enzyme defects are all autosomal recessive traits and show a wide range in frequency of occurrence: 21-hydroxylase deficiency is the most common form, occurring in 90–95% of CAH cases. Approximately 5% of CAH cases are owed to deficiency of 11β-hydroxylase, while deficiencies of 3-hydroxysteroid dehydrogenase, 17/20-lyase, 17-hydroxylase, and StAR protein are very rare.

Defects in 11β-hydroxylation result in virilizing congenital adrenal hyperplasia that is often accompanied by hypertension. Elevated serum levels of deoxycorticosterone (DOC) and 11-deoxycortisol (S) exert a net mineralocorticoid effect, altering renal function and causing sodium retention and volume expansion. Virilization and hypertension are the prominent clinical features of 11β-hydroxylase deficiency. Accumulation of precursors increases substrate availability for ACTH-stimulated 17,20-lyase activity in the unimpeded androgen pathways, and adrenal androgen secretion is increased. Development of the female external genitalia is affected *in utero* by excess fetal adrenal androgens, resulting in ambiguous external genitalia (female pseudohermaphroditism) in all cases. Postnatally, continued excessive adrenal androgen production results in premature and inappropriate somatic development in both boys and girls: progressive penile/clitoral enlargement, appearance of axillary hair, pubic hair, and facial hair, acne, deepening of voice, and rapid skeletal growth. Without treatment, early epiphyseal maturation results in short stature.

Hypertension is a less consistent feature than virilization in 11β-hydroxylase deficiency. It is usually not identified until later in childhood or in adolescence, although its appearance in an infant 3 months of age has been documented.[4] In addition, hypertension correlates variably with biochemical values.[5,6] Potassium depletion develops concomitantly with sodium retention, but hypokalemia is variable. Renin production is suppressed secondary to steroid-induced sodium retention and volume expansion. Aldosterone production is low secondary to low serum [K^+] and low plasma renin. The degree of hyporeninemia may vary widely, and in at least two reported cases has been absent.[7]

Biochemically, 11β-hydroxylase is responsible in the ZF for the conversion of 11-deoxycortisol (compound S) to cortisol in the 17-hydroxy pathway, and, in the 17-deoxy pathway, for the conversion of deoxycorticosterone (DOC) to corticosterone (compound B). In the zona glomerulosa (ZG), the conversion of DOC to B is one of a number of related conversions, which in series yield aldosterone, the regulated product of this zone. As well as being 11β-hydroxylated to B, DOC can be instead 18-hydroxylated to 18-hydroxy-11-deoxycorticosterone (18-OHDOC), which then can be 11-hydroxylated to 18-hydroxycorticosterone (18-OHB). The final step of aldosterone synthesis, the 18-oxidation of 18-OHB, is catalyzed by the enzyme by aldosterone synthase (cytochrome P450aldo), which is an isoform of 11β-hydroxylase.

Chronic elevation of ACTH in response to low plasma cortisol results in increased synthesis and secretion of steroid intermediates proximal to the 11β-hydroxylase block and their non-11β-hydroxylated products.[8] These include 11β-hydroxylase substrates compound S (11-deoxycortisol), DOC, the S precursor 17-hydroxyprogesterone (17-OHP), and $^{4\text{-}}$androstenedione

(^{4}-A). In female infants with ambiguous genitalia, serum elevations of the S and DOC are characteristic of an 11-hydroxylase deficiency. Serum 17-OHP and its major urinary metabolite, pregnanetriol, are elevated, but not as greatly as in 21-hydroxylase deficiency CAH.

The significant mineralocorticoid potency of the steroid DOC was recognized early in clinical studies in which it was administered as an exogenous agent,[9] and thus the elevation of DOC in the plasma steroid profile is presumed to be central to the volume-expanded hypertension induced in 11-hydroxylase deficiency. It is not confirmed that DOC is the only factor in the development of hypertension, as blood pressure and DOC levels have not been well-correlated in patients.[10,11] Glucocorticoid administration provides cortisol function and normalizes ACTH, which in turn removes the drive for oversecretion of DOC—the adrenal secretion studies of New and Seaman showed that plasma DOC arises largely from the ZF—and in most cases brings about remission of hypertension. Serum DOC is thus the principal steroid index of the 11β-hydroxylase defect and its normalization the indicator of its hormonal control.

Endocrine challenge/suppression studies undertaken to evaluate zonal differences in 11b-hydroxylase deficiency have determined that the ZF exhibits reduced 11b-hydroxylation and 18-hydroxylation, while both functions appear to be spared in the ZG.[12] This explains the effect of glucocorticoid treatment, which by diminishing secretion of DOC and producing natriuresis and diuresis, restores the plasma volume to a normal value, bringing plasma renin up to levels able to stimulate aldosterone production via the separate 11b-/18-hydroxylating system of the ZG.

MOLECULAR GENETICS OF 11β-HYDROXYLASE

The adrenal steroid 11β-hydroxylase is the enzyme cytochrome P450c11. Whereas for a time it was thought that the terminal steps of aldosterone synthesis were also catalyzed by the identical molecular species of cytochrome P450,[13] it has now been established that there are two closely related isoforms, cytochrome $P450_{C11}$ and cytochrome P450aldo, the products of two homologous genes,[14] CYP11B1 (encoding the 11-hydroxylase isoform)[15] and CYP11B2 (encoding the aldosterone synthase isoform),[16,17] located about 30 kb apart on the long arm of chromosome 8.

Steroid 11β-hydroxylase deficiency is the result of mutations affecting the type or expression of the CYP11B1 gene.[18–20] More than 30 mutations have been identified in patients with 11b-OHD.[21] The majority of mutations are random point mutations, although gene conversions between CYP11B1 and CYP11B2 have been found.[18,22,23] Worldwide, 11b-OHD occurs in approximately 1 in 100,000 births, with a significantly higher incidence in Jewish families of North African origin, particularly from Morocco and Tunisia.[6,24]

APPARENT MINERALOCORTICOID EXCESS (AME)

Apparent mineralocorticoid excess (AME) was first defined as a syndrome in 1977 by New and coworkers in their clinical evaluation of a patient with an extremely unusual endocrine profile. In this case (a young female child, member of the Zuñi tribe of the Southwest of the United States) were found hypertension, significant hypokalemia, metabolic alkalosis, and suppressed renin but with low serum aldosterone and very low secretion rates of all standardly assayable corticosteroids, in spite of which there were no signs of adrenal insufficiency.[25] Following observations of possible biochemical defects in the clearance of cortisol, and numerous attempts to identify an unknown steroid acting potently both as a glucocorticoid and a mineralocorticoid, it was by 1983 postulated that cortisol itself was the hypertensinogenic agent in this syndrome.[26] Molecular genetic studies of AME patients revealed mutations in the locus for the gene *HSD11B2*, which encodes the type-2 kidney isoform of the 11β-hydroxysteroid dehydrogenase (11β-HSD) enzyme.[27] This enzyme converts cortisol to cortisone, and is essential for separation of the physiological actions of cortisol and aldosterone.

Apparent mineralocorticoid excess is difficult to treat and shows a high degree of morbidity/mortality.[28] Diagnostic features include severe hypertension, failure to thrive, and persistent polydipsia and polyuria. Biochemical profiles show metabolic alkalosis and severe hypokalemia. Plasma renin activity (PRA) is low, suggesting a volume-expanded type of hypertension, responding to dietary sodium restriction. All steroid levels, including aldosterone, are very low. The hypertension in this disorder is very severe, leading often to early end organ damage, and with significant mortality. The biochemical diagnosis can be made by measuring the ratio of cortisol to cortisone, or the ratio of their metabolites. A more definitive diagnosis can be made by measuring the level of tritiated water in plasma samples when 11-tritiated cortisol is injected. In one study in two patients with AME, there was little or no measurable production of tritiated water, while in normal subjects and heterozygotes, 65–80 percent of the tritiated label appears as tritiated water.[29] Treatment consists of mineralocorticoid receptor blockade with spironolactone, usually in quite high doses, resulting in an initial lowering of arterial blood sugar and increase in serum potassium.

PATHOPHYSIOLOGY AND MOLECULAR GENETICS OF AME

For many years it has been known that the root of the licorice plant *Glycyrrhizae glabra* can induce sodium retention with elevated blood pressure and potassium wasting. Clinical studies showed that the presence of corticosteroids was necessary to elicit this hypertensinogenic effect since administration of licorice root extracts to patients with Addison's disease was without effect. Also, studies of the type I and type II steroid receptors revealed for the type I receptor, the classical mineralocorticoid receptor (MR), that the isolated receptor had as great an intrinsic affinity *in vitro* for cortisol as for aldosterone. How then, it was asked, could aldosterone, present in the plasma in levels 2–3 orders of magnitude less than glucocorticoids, access the MR, even allowing for its much lesser protein-bound and increased unbound (active) fraction?

An answer to this question and explanation for the origin of the excess mineralocorticoid steroid effect in AME came with a new mechanistic postulate, that selectivity of mineralocorticoid action is determined not by the MR ligand-binding site, which is in fact nonspecific, but by an intracellular enzyme that systematically inactivates unintended candidate steroids (glucocorticoids) and thereby protects the MR from saturation. The enzyme 11β-hydroxysteroid dehydrogenase type 2 (11β-HSD2), active in the collecting duct cells of the kidneys, catalyzes the conversion of cortisol (F) to cortisone (E).[30] The MR receptor affinity for cortisone is much less than for cortisol because stereoscopic factors do not permit cortisone to bind. This action of the 11β-HSD2 enzyme forms the mechanism by which normal subjects are protected from cortisol intoxication. Failure of this mechanism occurs in AME patients, as they have a deficiency of enzyme 11β-HSD2. Excess serum cortisol results and saturates the mineralocorticoid receptor, causing sodium retention and volume expansion that suppresses plasma renin and aldosterone secretion. Prolonged availability of cortisol, owing an extended half-life, results in ACTH suppression and, thus, decreased adrenal cortical secretion.

In 1994, the gene for 11β-hydroxysteroid dehydrogenase type 2, *HSD11B2*, was cloned and mapped to human chromosome 16.[31] Shortly thereafter, genetic analysis of a family with AME-affected members identified a mutation (R337C) in the HSD11B2 gene of two of the three sibs suffering from AME.[32] These patients, as is true with all but two AME patients, appear to be homozygous for one of the 19 identified mutations.[33] Though identified mutations causing AME are different, they share the following features: (1) With one exception, the mutations all occur in the coding region of the HSD11B2 gene; (2) the mutations segregate with the disease; (3) the tested parents are heterozygous; (4) unaffected siblings are either heterozygous or homozygous unaffected; and (5) consanguinity and identity by descent are increased as expected in an autosomal recessive disorder.

A second AME type has been observed in one patient, in which defective steroid 11-oxidation, which was clearly shown by altered excretory THF + alloTHF/THE ratios initially in all AME patients, was in fact normal. A homozygous mutation (P227L) in exon 4 of HSD11B2was found in this biochemically distinct patient with mild hypertension.[34] The parents of the patient with mild AME are consanguineous Mennonites of Prussian descent.

A study of this Mennonite community in Kansas revealed a heterozygote frequency of 2.4% for the P2271 mutation.[35] Just as identification of the rare hypertensive disorder AME (as indeed for the other adrenocortical low-renin disorders earlier discussed) has opened speculation on little-understood aspects of steroid hormonal functions, further characterization of this disorder, and especially the mild form, will increase understanding of physiological processes of low-renin hypertension.

SUMMARY

Early identification and treatment of hypertension will prevent organ damage and minimize the systemic vascular changes that progress into the resistant picture of low-renin hypertension. Understanding the pathogenesis of CAH owing to 11β-hydroxylase deficiency and AME is of the utmost importance. Specific therapy is best, which means early identification of the underlying cause. For this to be done, these relatively uncommon disorders must be investigated as carefully and completely as possible by study of individual cases. Further elucidation of endocrine origins and course of development of hypertension will improve therapy and benefit affected children

ACKNOWLEDGMENTS

We wish to express our appreciation to Andrea Putnam for her editorial assistance in the preparation of this manuscript.

Significant sections of the work on which the data are reported herein were supported by United States PHS Grant HD00072 and Clinical Research Center Grant RR 06020.

REFERENCES

1. WILLIAMS, R., S. HUNT, P. HOPKINS, *et al.* 1994. Kidney Intl **45:** S57–S64.
2. NEW, M.I. & L.S. LEVINE. 1973. *In* Advances in Human Genetics. H. Harris, & K. Hirschhorn, Eds. Vol. 4: 251–326. Plenum. New York.
3. NEW, M.I., P.C. WHITE, S. PANG, *et al.* 1989. *In* The Metabolic Basis of Inherited Disease. C.R. Scriver *et al.*, Eds. :1881–1917. McGraw-Hill. New York.
4. MIMOUNI, M., H. KAUFMAN, A. ROITMAN, *et al.* 1985. Eur. J. Pediatr. **143:** 231–233.
5. ROSLER, A., E. LEIBERMAN & J. SACK. 1982. Hormone Res. **16:** 133.
6. ROSLER, A. & E. LEIBERMAN. 1984. *In* Adrenal Diseases in Childhood: Pathophysiologic and Clinical Aspects M.I. New & L.S. Levine, Eds. Vol. 13: 47–71. S. Karger, Basel.

7. NEW, M.I., R.L. NEMERY, D.M. CHOW, et al. 1989. In The Adrenal and Hypertension: From Cloning to Clinic. E.G. Biglieri, et al., Eds. :323–343. Raven Press. Tokyo.
8. EBERLEIN, W. & A. BONGIOVANNI. 1956. J. Biol. Chem. **223:** 85.
9. PERERA, G., A. KNOWLTON, A. LOWELL & R. LOEB. 1944. JAMA **125:** 1030.
10. GREEN, O.C., C.J. MIGEON & L. WILKINS. 1960. J. Clin. Endocrinol. Metab. **20:** 929–946.
11. GLENTHOJ, A., M.D. NIELSEN & J. STARUP. 1980. Acta Endocrinol (Copenh.) **93:** 94–99.
12. LEVINE, L.S., W. RAUH, K. GOTTESDIENER, et al. 1980. J. Clin. Endocrinol. Metab. **50:** 258–63.
13. YANAGIBASHI, K., M. HANIU, J. SHIVELY, et al. 1986. J. Biol. Chem. **261:** 3556–3562.
14. MORNET, E., J. DUPONT, A. VITEK & P. WHITE. 1989. J. Biol. Chem. **264:** 20961–20967.
15. CHUA, S., P. SZABO, A. VITEK, et al. 1987. Proc. Natl. Acad. Sci. USA **84:** 7193–7197.
16. CURNOW, K., M. TUSIE-LUNA, L. PASCOE, et al. 1991. Mol. Endocrinol. **5:** 1513–1522.
17. KAWAMOTO, T., Y. MITSUUCHI, K. TODA, et al. 1992. Proc. Natl. Acad. Sci. USA **89:** 1458–1462.
18. WHITE, P. C., J. DUPONT, M.I. NEW, et al. 1991. J. Clin. Invest. **87:** 1664–1667.
19. CURNOW, K.M., L. SLUTSKER, J. VITEK, et al. 1993. Proc. Natl. Acad. Sci. USA **90:** 4552–4556.
20. SKINNER, C. & G. RUMSBY. 1994. Hum. Mol. Genet. **3:** 377–378.
21. KRAWCZAK, M. & D.N. COOPER. 1997. Trends Genet. **13:** 121–122.
22. MERKE, D.P., T. TAJIMA, A. CHHABRA, et al. 1998. J. Clin. Endocrinol. Metab. **83:** 270–273.
23. MULATERO, P., K.M. CURNOW, B. AUPETIT-FAISANT, et al. 1998. J. Clin. Endocrinol. Metab. **83:** 3996–4001.
24. ZACHMANN, M., D. TASSINARI & A. PRADER. 1983. J. Endocrinol. Metab. **56:** 222–229.
25. NEW, M.I., L.S. LEVINE, E.G. BIGLIERI, et al. 1977. J. Clin. Endocrinol. Metab. **44:** 924–33.
26. NEW, M.I., S.E. OBERFIELD, R.M. CAREY, et al. 1982. In Endocrinology of Hypertension, Serono Symposia No. 50. F. Mantero, et al., Eds. :85–101. Academic Press. New York.
27. STEWART, P.M., Z.S. KROZOWSKI, A. GUPTA, et al. 1996. Lancet **347:** 88–91.
28. DOWNEY, M.K., L. RIDDICK & M.I. NEW. 1987. In Program and Abstracts, American Society of Hypertension Second World Congress on Biologically Active Atrial Peptides, New York.
29. ULICK, S., L.S. LEVINE, P. GUNCZLER, et al. 1979. J. Clin. Endocrinol. Metab. **49:** 757–764.
30. LAKSHMI, V. & C. MONDER. 1985. Endocrinology **116:** 552–560.
31. ALBISTON, A.L., V.R. OBEYESEKERE, R.E. SMITH & Z.S. KROZOWSKI. 1994. Mol. Cell. Endocrinol. **105:** R11–17.
32. WILSON, R.C., M.D. HARBISON, Z.S. KROZOWSKI, et al. 1995. J. Clin. Endocrinol. Metab. **80:** 3145–3150.
33. WILSON, R., S. NIMKARN & M.I. NEW. 2001. Trends Endocrinol. Metab. **12:** 104–111.

34. WILSON, R.C., S. DAVE–SHARMA, J. WEI, *et al.* 1998. Proc. Natl. Acad. Sci, USA **95:** 10200–10205.
35. UGRASBUL, F., T. WIENS, P. RUBINSTEIN, *et al.* 1999. Prevalence of mild apparent mineralocorticoid excess in Mennonites. J. Clin. Endocrinl. Metab. 84: 4735–4738.
36. NEW, M.I. & P.C. WHITE. 1995. *In* Genetic and Molecular Biological Aspects of Endocrine Disease. :526. Ballière Tindall. London.

The Diagnosis and Management of Endocrine Tumors Causing Hypertension in Children

KURT D. NEWMAN AND TODD PONSKY

Departments of Surgery and Pediatrics, Children's Hospital and George Washington University School of Medicine, Washington, D.C., USA

ABSTRACT: In contrast to that in adults, hypertension in children is frequently amenable to surgical therapy. With advancing techniques in imaging, surgery, and anesthesia, the outcomes of surgery are excellent for children with endocrine tumors causing hypertension.

KEYWORDS: pheochromocytoma; endocrine tumors; hypertension; children

Hypertension is becoming increasingly recognized as a public health issue for children and adolescents. The prevalence of hypertension in children is estimated to be approximately 1–3%. In a significant number of children, hypertension results from an endocrine tumor. The management of children with hypertension due to endocrine tumors has evolved owing to progress in genetics, imaging, anesthesia and surgical technique.

Although there is a wide spectrum of etiologic factors in childhood hypertension, the causes are more often amenable to surgery than in adults. These causative factors include renal artery stenosis and coarctation of the aorta, hyperthyroidism, adrenogenital syndrome, Conn's and Cushing's syndromes, brain tumors, and frequently essential hypertension. Tumors constitute an important source of hypertension in children, not only from a biologic viewpoint, but also because they are often treatable with concomitant resolution of the hypertension. Patients with malignant tumors can present with hypertension, most notably Wilms' tumor and neuroblastoma. The mechanism for hypertension from neuroblastoma is either through renal artery compression

---

Address for correspondence: Kurt D. Newman, M.D., Children's National Medical Center, 111 Michigan Avenue, N.W., Washington, D.C., 20010. Voice: 202-884-2151.
knewman@cnmc.org

or catecholamine secretion. Resection of the tumor usually resolves the high blood pressure.

Primary hyperaldosteronism is an unusual source of hypertension in children. Adrenocortical hyperplasia is the most common cause. Adrenocortical carcinomas are rare causes of high blood pressure, but are very invasive tumors in children and require aggressive surgery. When a functional adenoma is identified, the treatment is complete excision.

Pheochromocytomas are responsible for approximately 1% of non-essential hypertension in children. The tumors arise from chromaffin cells in the sympathetic-adrenal system. Thirty percent of children will have an extra-adrenal pheochromocytoma. Sites may be in the bladder, brain, thorax, neck, paraganglia, or organ of Zuckerkandl. Ten percent of all pheochromocytomas occur in children. The presentation is most commonly at 8 or 9 years of age, and almost 10 percent will have a family history because of the association of multiple endocrine neoplasia (MEN) syndromes.

Children with pheochromocytoma commonly present with throbbing headaches, pallor with flushing, fever, sweating, nausea, or weight loss despite a huge appetite. Frequently they will have sustained hypertension related to the ratio of norepinephrine to epinephrine. This is different from the adult situation, where the hypertension is usually intermittent. Less common symptoms are visual problems, pain, heat intolerance, and swelling.

The genetics of pheochromocytoma has received much study. Four percent of the tumors are associated with genetic abnormalities of neural crest derivatives. Among the heritable causes of pheochromocytoma are MEN-2A and -2B, Von Hippel–Landau syndrome, neurofibromatosis, and paraganglionic syndromes. In MEN-2 syndromes the pheochromocytoma is often associated with medullary carcinoma of the thyroid, parathyroid tumors, and mucosal neuromas. Approximately 50% of patients with MEN-2A will develop a pheochromocytoma, although the tumors in MEN-2B are more aggressive.

Screening and early identification have played a major role in the improved survival of children with pheochromocytoma. Children in families known to be at risk for pheochromocytoma can be screened with periodic retroperitoneal imaging and/or measurement of plasma metanephrines or 24-hour urine collections for catecholamines and metanephrines. If MEN is a consideration, the children will be screened for the RET mutation. If positive for this mutation, the children will undergo thyroidectomy to prevent and treat medullary carcinoma of the thyroid. They also undergo periodic screening for pheochromocytoma. However, the most cost-effective strategy for screening remains to be identified.

Once a pheochromocytoma is suspected in a child, careful and expeditious management is essential to prevent complications or even death. Frequently the child is admitted to the hospital for inpatient hypertension control and adrenergic blockade. Preoperative localization of the tumor is critical particularly because of the high incidence of bilaterality in children as well as the possibility of an extra-adrenal site. The risk of these presentations is much higher than in the adult patients. CT scan or MRI is essential and commonly MIBG scans provide important anatomic or functional information. The precision of preoperative scanning has permitted the addition of techniques such as laparoscopy and adrenal-sparing surgery to the armamentarium of the surgeon.

The perioperative and anesthetic management of children with pheochromocytoma has become extremely successful. Sudden death was at one time frequent in these children, but is now rarely seen. The children receive both alpha- and beta-adrenergic blockade. They are admitted for preoperative hydration. Intraoperatively they are monitored with arterial and central lines and urinary catheters. The pharmacological management of intraoperative and postoperative hypertension and pain has become quite sophisticated and effective.

Surgical treatment is directed toward complete resection of the tumor, which classically has meant total removal of the involved adrenal gland. Some surgeons advocate adrenal-sparing surgery because of the risk of adrenal insufficiency if the contralateral adrenal requires removal. However in children this risk is balanced by the possibility of carcinoma in the tumor. Therefore complete resection is still advocated for most children. Laparoscopic approaches to resection have become popular due to the smaller incisions and improved recovery times for patients with this approach. Success has been reported in children with single-sided tumors. Key surgical principles are early ligation of the venous drainage to control catecholamine release as well as careful extraction of the tumor to prevent tumor spillage. Advocates of laparoscopy cite the ability to inspect the entire abdomen and retroperitoneum as additional advantages of this approach.

Cancer occurs in fewer than 6 percent of childhood cases of pheochromocytoma. Malignancy is very difficult to differentiate histologically so the biologic behavior of the tumor determines the classification. Children who experience recurrence will usually develop recurrent symptoms within a year of diagnosis. The presence of extra-adrenal cells in tissues where chromaffin cells are not normally found indicates metastatic disease. The efficacy of chemotherapy continues to be studied.

The success of management of children with endocrine tumors correlates with the scientific advances in genetics, imaging, pharmacology, and surgical technique. The integration of this new knowledge with clinical care now permits most children to have safe and effective treatment of these tumors. Because of sensitive screening and accurate imaging the tumors are identified early and located precisely. The anesthetic management and evolution of surgical technique have resulted in superb outcomes. Long-term follow up studies are in progress to confirm the sustained success of treatment.

REFERENCES

1. BRANDI, M.L. *et al.* 2001. Consensus guidelines for diagnosis and therapy of MEN type1 and type 2. J. Clin. Endocrinol. Metab. **86:** 5658–5671.
2. GAGEL, R.F., A.H. TASHJIAN, JR., T. CUMMINGS, *et al.* 1988. The clinical outcome of prospective screening for multiple endocrine neoplasia type 2a: an 18 year experience. N. Engl. J. Med. 318: 478–484.
3. CASANOVA, S., M. ROSENBERG-BOURGIN, D. FARKAS, *et al.* 1993. Phaeochromocytoma in multiple endocrine neoplasia type 2A: a survey of 100 cases. Clin. Endocrinol. (Oxf.) **38:** 531–537.
4. LAIRMORE, T.C., D.W. BALL, S.B. BAYLIN, *et al.* 1993. Management of pheochromocytomas in patients with multiple endocrine neoplasia type 2 syndromes. Ann. Surg. **217:** 595–601.
5. GAGNER, M., G. BRETON, D. PHARAND, *et al.* 1996. Is laparoscopic adrenalectomy indicated for pheochromocytomas? Surgery **120:** 1076–1079.
6. LEE, J.E., S.A. CURLEY, R.F. GAGEL, *et al.* 1996. Cortical-sparing adrenalectomy for patients with bilateral pheochromocytoma. Surgery **120:** 1064–1070.
7. KINNEY, M.A., M.E. WARNER, J.A. VANHEERDEN, *et al.* 2000. Perianesthetic risks and outcomes of pheochromocytomas and paraganglionic resection. Anesth. Analg. **91:** 1118–1123.
8. RAEBURN, C.D. & R.C. MCINTYRE, JR. 2000. Laparoscopic approach to adrenal and endocrine pancreatic tumors. Surg. Clin. N. Amer. **80:** 1427–1441.
9. LIOU, L.S. & R. KAY. 2000. Adrenocortical carcinoma in children: review and recent innovations. Urol. Clin. N. Amer. **27:** 403–421.
10. NEUMANN, H.P., B.U. BENDER, M. REINCKE, *et al.* 1999. Adrenal-sparing surgery for pheochromocytoma. Br. J. Surg. **86:** 94–97.
11. GOLDSTEIN, R.E., J.A. O'NEILL, JR., G.W. HOLCOMB, 3RD, *et al.* 2001. Clinical experience over 48 years with pheochromocytoma. Ann. Surg. **229:** 753–764.
12. CIFTCI, A.O., F.C. TANYEL, M.E. SENOCAK, *et al.* 2001. Pheochromocytoma in children. J. Pediat. Surg. **36:** 447–452.
13. REDDY, V.S., J.A. O'NEILL, JR., G.W. HOLCOMB, 3RD, *et al.* 2000. Twenty-five year surgical experience with pheochromocytoma in children. Am. Surgeon **66:** 1085–1091.
14. ROSS, J.H. 2000. Pheochromocytoma: special considerations in children. Urol. Clin. N. Amer. **27:** 393–402.
15. GRUNWALD, Z. & K.E. MEYERS. 1999. Hypertension in Infants and Children: Anesthesia and Hypertension. Anesthesiology Clinics of North America, Vol. **17.** W.B. Saunders. Philadelphia, PA.

The Role of PET in Localization of Neuroendocrine and Adrenocortical Tumors

BARBRO ERIKSSON,[a] MATS BERGSTRÖM,[b] ANDERS SUNDIN,[c] CLAES JUHLIN,[d] HÅKAN ÖRLEFORS,[a] KJELL ÖBERG,[a] AND BENGT LÅNGSTRÖM[b]

[a]*Department of Medical Sciences,* [b]*Uppsala University PET-Centre, and Departments of* [c]*Radiology and* [d]*Surgery, University Hospital, S-751 85 Uppsala, Sweden*

ABSTRACT: Positron emission tomography (PET) supplies a range of labeled compounds to be used for the characterization of tumor biochemistry. Some of these have proved to be of value for clinical diagnosis, treatment follow up, and clinical research. The first routinely used PET tracer in oncology, ^{18}F-labeled deoxyglucose (FDG), was successfully used for diagnosis of cancer, reflecting increased expression of glucose transporter in cancerous tissue. This tracer, however, usually does not show sufficient uptake in well-differentiated tumors such as neuroendocrine tumors. We developed a tracer more specific to neuroendocrine tumors—the serotonin precursor 5-hydroxytryptophan (5-HTP) labeled with ^{11}C—and demonstrated increased uptake and irreversible trapping of this tracer in carcinoid tumors. The uptake was so selective and the resolution was so high that we could detect more liver and lymph node metastases with PET than with CT or octreotide scintigraphy. To further improve the method, especially to reduce the high renal excretion of the tracer producing streaky artifacts in the area of interest, we introduced premedication by the decarboxylase inhibitor carbidopa, leading to a six-fold decreased renal excretion while the tumor uptake increased three-fold, hence improving the visualization of the tumors.

^{11}C-labeled L-DOPA was evaluated as an alternative tracer, especially for endocrine pancreatic tumors, which usually do not demonstrate enhanced urinary serotonin metabolites. However, only half of the EPTs, mainly functioning tumors, could be detected with L-DOPA. Instead 5-HTP seems to be a universal tracer for EPT and foregut carcinoids. With new, more sensitive PET cameras, larger field of view and procedures for whole-body coverage, the PET examination with 5-HTP is now routinely

Address for correspondence: Barbro Eriksson, M.D., Ph.D., Clinic for Endocrine Oncology, Department of Medical Sciences, University Hospital, SE-751 85 Uppsala, Sweden. Voice: 46-18-6112716.
barbro.Eriksson@medsci.uu.se

performed as reduced whole-body PET examinations with coverage of the thorax and abdomen. With this method we have been able to visualize small neuroendocrine lesions in the pancreas and thorax (e.g., ACTH-producing bronchial carcinoids) not detectable by any other method, including octreotide scintigraphy, MRI, and CT. Another tracer, the 11β-hydroxylase inhibitor, metomidate labeled with ^{11}C, was developed to simplify diagnosis and follow-up of patients with incidentalomas. A large series of patients with incidentally found adrenal masses have been investigated and so far all lesions of adrenocortical origin have been easily identified because of exceedingly high uptake of ^{11}C-metomidate, whereas noncortical lesions showed very low uptake. In addition, adrenocortical cancer shows high uptake, suggesting that this PET tracer can be used for staging purposes.

KEYWORDS: positron emission tomography; neuroendocrine tumors; 5-hydroxytryptophan (5-HTP); L-dihyroxyphenylalanine (L-DOPA); metomidate; whole-body PET

NEUROENDOCRINE TUMORS

Introduction

Neuroendocrine tumors derive from endocrine cells; they usually contain secretory granulae and have the capacity to produce biogenic amines and polypeptide hormones. As early as 20 years ago, Pearse presented the so-called APUD-concept based on the observation that certain cells have the capacity to take up and decarboxylate amine precursors (*a*mine *p*recursor *u*ptake and *d*ecarboxylation) such as 5-hydroxytryptophan (5-HTP) and L-dihydroxyphenylalanine (L-DOPA). Tumors derived from these cells were consequently called APUDomas.[1]

Carcinoids are usually classified according to embryonic origin into foregut, midgut, and hindgut, a classification which is still relevant because these different tumors have different tendencies to metastasize and have different symptomatology.[2] The midgut carcinoid, usually originating from cells in the small intestine, has a relatively high tendency to metastasize via local lymph nodes to the liver, and most patients have liver metastases at diagnosis. At this stage most patients present the carcinoid syndrome, including symptoms of flush, diarrhea, bronchoconstriction, and right-sided heart failure, caused by overproduction of substances such as serotonin and tachykinins.[3] Serotonin is produced by the carcinoid tumor cells via two enzymatic steps: first, tryptophan is 5-hydroxylated to 5-HTP, which in turn is decarboxylated to serotonin (5-hydroxytryptamine or 5-HT) by aromatic amino acid decarboxylase (AADC). Serotonin circulating in the blood is predominantly bound to platelets. Unbound serotonin is oxidatively amidated to 5-hydroxyindoleacetic acid (5-HIAA). 5-HIAA is excreted in the urine and has until now been one of the most important tumor markers for diagnosis and treatment follow up in carcinoid patients.[4]

Carcinoids of foregut origin, such as bronchial and gastric carcinoids, have a lesser tendency to metastasize to the liver, and they infrequently produce serotonin because of a lack of aromatic amino acid decarboxylase. Instead, other substances are produced, such as pancreatic polypeptide, human chorionic gonadotropin alpha, adrenocorticotropin (ACTH), and histamine. Hindgut carcinoids metastasize in about 20% of cases and rarely present hormonal symptoms or elevation of U-5-HIAA despite the content of peptides and hormones in the tumors.

Endocrine pancreatic tumors (EPT) are classified according to hormone production and associated symptoms into the following clinical syndromes: insulinomas, gastrinomas, watery-diarrhea–hypokalemia–achlorhydria (WDHA), glucagonomas, and somatostatinomas. In malignant tumors, mixed syndromes are common due to multiple hormone production from the tumors. About one-third of EPTs are hormonally silent despite their content and production of hormones, and these tumors are called nonfunctioning tumors. EPTs can also be part of the multiple endocrine neoplasia (MEN) 1 syndrome, in which multiple pancreatic tumors are almost always found.

Diagnostic Methods in Neuroendocrine Tumors

The diagnostic methods that are currently available, including CT, ultrasonography, and MRI, often fail to localize small primary tumors, for example, insulinomas and gastrinomas. Selective angiography has often been used to localize small tumors, but this procedure is invasive and often falsely positive. Endoscopic ultrasonography is a new technique, which is relatively sensitive but not available in all centers. Ultrasonography performed intraoperatively has shown the greatest sensitivity, but it is always of advantage to the surgeon to know the localization of the tumor preoperatively.

Octreotide scintigraphy (Octreoscan), based on the presence of somatostatin receptors (SSTR 1-5) in 80–90% of neuroendocrine tumors, is nowadays a routine investigation tool in all newly diagnosed patients with neuroendocrine gastrointestinal tumors.[5] Diagnostically, it has represented a great improvement because it is a whole-body examination and the patient's disease can be staged; furthermore, it is a predictive test for sensitivity to somatostatin analogue treatment.[6] The method may have problems in localizing small tumors and such tumors that lack somatostatin receptor, for example, 50% of insulinomas.

Medical Treatment

Surgery is the treatment of choice if feasible, but the majority of patients have multiple liver metastases at diagnosis, which means that they are beyond surgical cure. Medical treatment is then warranted, and during the last 10–20 years several therapeutic options have been developed. Alpha-interferon (IFN) and somatostatin analogues and combinations of them are established therapies in both carcinoids and EPT; they can control hormonal symptoms by reducing circulating hormone levels for extended periods of time.[7,8] In a small group of patients (10–15%), a significant reduction in tumor size (>50%) can be noted, but in the majority of patients the tumor size remains unchanged on CT or MRI. However, during IFN-treatment the number of tumor cells is reduced and replaced by fibrosis.[9] Furthermore, high-dose somatostatin analogue treatment induces apoptosis in the tumors of responding patients.[10] These phenomena cannot be detected by conventional radiological methods. Specific chemotherapy with streptozocin in combination with 5-fluorouracil/doxorubicin can be effective in malignant EPT and produces biochemical and/or radiological responses in 50% of patients with a median duration of two years.[7] In contrast, midgut carcinoids have been rather resistant to various combinations of chemotherapeutic drugs.[8] However, in a subset of carcinoid tumors, particularly foregut carcinoids (lung, thymus), the combination of cisplatin plus etoposide has produced remarkable remissions.[11] This is true also for anaplastic EPT.

PET EXAMINATIONS WITH ^{11}C-LABELED 5-HTP

For visualization of tumors in general, the prime PET tracer has been FDG. At our Centre, PET with FDG failed to show enhanced accumulation in a small number of patients with neuroendocrine tumors. Similar observations were made comparing the value of FDG-PET to octreotide scintigraphy in the imaging of neuroendocrine tumors.[12] Increased uptake of FDG could only be seen in a small number of less-differentiated neuroendocrine tumors with high proliferative activity and without somatostatin receptors (negative octreotide scintigraphy).

Neuroendocrine tumors have previously been classified as APUDomas, based on Pearse's old characterization of amine precursor uptake and decarboxylation. Because increased serotonin synthesis is one of the diagnostic criteria of the carcinoid syndrome, it appeared logical to use a labeled precursor for serotonin as a tracer. In a pilot trial, tryptophan labeled with ^{11}C was used, but did not show high uptake in carcinoid liver metastases. However, 5-HTP ^{11}C-labeled in the β-position showed a very high uptake in the tumors as compared to normal organs, including the liver (FIG. 1). Kinetic analysis of the tracer uptake indicated irreversible trapping of the tracer in the tumors.[13] In further PET studies using specific-positioned labeling of 5-HTP in the β and carboxyl positions, the process of uptake and rapid decarboxylation of the tracer to serotonin was demonstrated.[14]

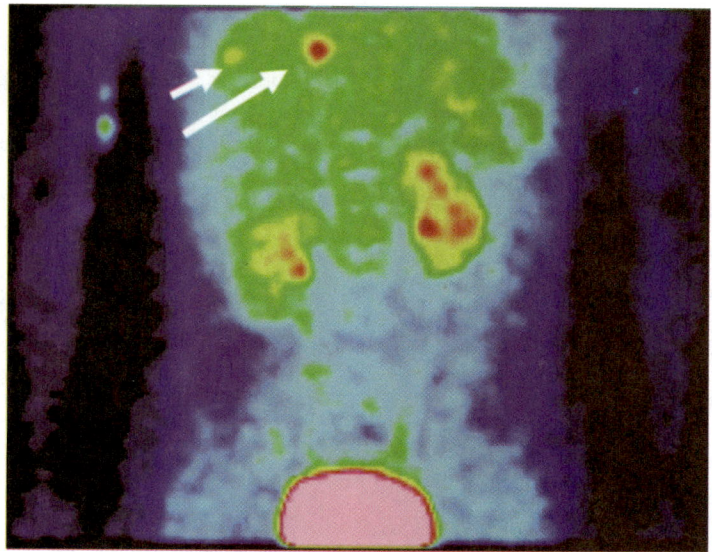

FIGURE 1. Whole-body PET with ^{11}C-labeled 5-HTP, demonstrating an ectopic adrenocorticotropin (ACTH)-producing bronchial carcinoid with metastases to the lung.

Visualization of Tumors

In a first study, 18 consecutive patients with neuroendocrine gastrointestinal tumors (midgut 14, foregut 1, hindgut 1) were examined.[13] All patients except two (1 EPT and 1 hindgut carcinoid) had elevations of U-5-HIAA. All patients, as well as those patients with normal U-5-HIAA, showed significantly increased uptake of the tracer in tumorous tissue (FIG. 2). More lesions could be detected with PET in comparison with those of CT. The selective and high uptake in tumor tissue compared to surrounding normal tissue (high tumor-to-background ratio) produced a very good tumor visibility. The initial optimistic results have been confirmed in more than 200 PET studies in patients with neuroendocrine tumors.

Pharmacological Modulation of Tracer Uptake

In most patients, a high concentration of radioactivity was observed in the renal pelvis due to the excretion of the tracer in the urine. Often this very high radioactivity produced streaky artifacts in the area of interest, which made the interpretation of images difficult. Studies were done in rats using different drugs to modulate the relative uptake in different organs, and it was found that decarboxylase inhibitors that block the peripheral amino-acid decarboxylase

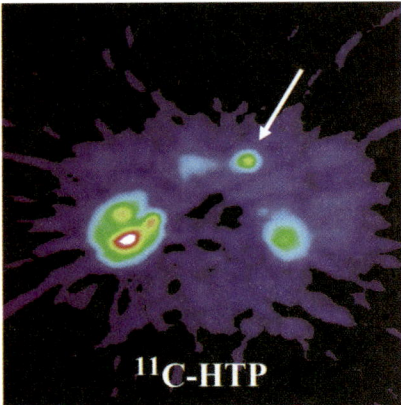 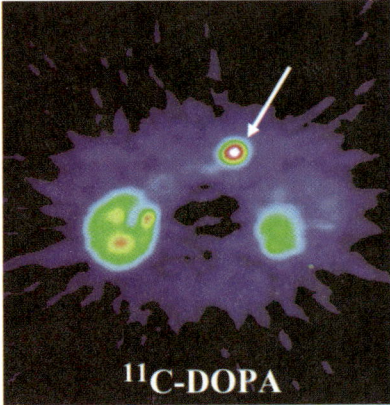

FIGURE 2. Patient with a nonfunctioning endocrine pancreatic tumor, examined both with ^{11}C-labeled 5-HTP (*left*) and with ^{11}C-L-DOPA (*right*).

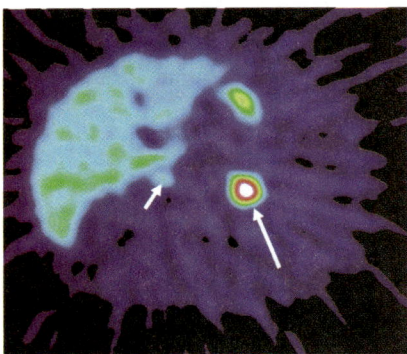 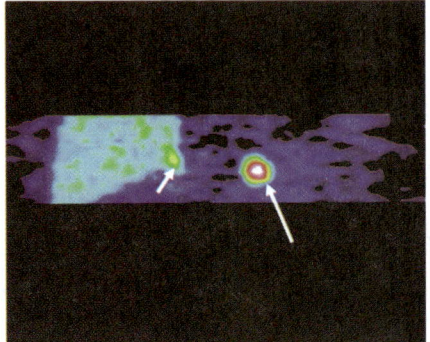

FIGURE 3. Transaxial (*left*) and coronal (*right*) images over the mid-abdomen showing highest uptake in an adrenal adenoma (*large arrow*), with lower uptake in normal adrenal gland (*small arrow*) and liver. Additional accumulation in the stomach.

could decrease the renal excretion significantly.[15] In a human trial, the radioactivity uptake in the renal pelvis decreased six-fold, and the tumoral uptake increased three-fold if the patient was pretreated with the decarboxylase inhibitor carbidopa. Peroral medication with carbidopa is therefore routinely used in association with PET studies with 5-HTP.

Therapy Monitoring

PET can also be used to study metabolic effects of treatment in the tumors.[12] Ten patients receiving different types of treatment (IFN, $n = 4$; IFN plus somatostatin analogue, $n = 2$; somatostatin analogue, $n = 4$) were followed before and at different time intervals after start of treatment (4 days, 3, 6, 12 months). When changes in the transport rate constant for the uptake of 5-HTP was compared to changes in U-5-HIAA during treatment, there was a >95% correlation using regression analysis. Thus, PET with 5-HTP may be a valuable complement for therapy monitoring, especially with tumors lacking tumor markers such as enhanced 5-HIAA and chromogranin A.

PET WITH ^{11}C-LABELED L-DIHYDROXYPHENYLALANINE (L-DOPA)

It is uncommon for patients with EPT to have elevation of U-5-HIAA as a sign of perturbed serotonin synthesis. It was therefore suggested that another amine precursor, L-DOPA, would be a valid tracer for these tumors. L-DOPA is an amino acid that is converted to the catecholamine dopamine by aromatic amino acid decarboxylase. In addition to its role as a precursor of adrenaline and noradrenaline, dopamine is a transmitter substance in the central nervous and peripheral nervous system. In this context, ^{11}C-labeled L-DOPA was applied as a tracer for dopamine synthesis.

Visualization of Tumors

Twenty-two consecutive patients with biochemically verified EPT were examined with ^{11}C-labeled L-DOPA.[16] Six patients had clinical symptoms of gastrinoma, four had glucagonoma, three insulinoma, six nonfunctioning tumors, one WDHA syndrome, and two had mixed functioning tumors. Six patients had the MEN 1 syndrome.

Increased uptake of the tracer in the primary tumor and metastases could be seen in 10 patients, mainly in functioning tumors (gastrinomas, glucagonomas) (FIG. 2). Nonfunctioning tumors were not detected using L-DOPA as a tracer. In addition, it was difficult to visualize small insulinomas, which had not been detected by any other preoperative radiological method, except by intraoperative ultrasonography.

^{11}F-Labeled L-Fluoro-DOPA

Although we do not have our own experience in the use of ^{18}F-labeled L-fluoro-DOPA, we have suggested that this tracer should be equivalent to ^{11}C-L-DOPA. Small differences do exist with respect to affinity to different enzymes. In other centers a few studies have been performed with positive results. The advantage of ^{18}F-L-fluoro-DOPA is its greater availability within the PET field and the longer half-life of the radionuclide; our own experience, however, suggests that ^{11}C-HTP has superior biological properties.

^{11}C-5-HTP AS A UNIVERSAL TRACER IN WHOLE-BODY PET

The observation in our previous study that several patients without elevation of U-5-HIAA had high uptake of 5-HTP in the tumors encouraged further exploration of this tracer as a valuable tracer for the diagnosis of neuroendocrine tumors. Furthermore, the possibility to modulate the uptake of 5-HTP with carbidopa has facilitated the performance of whole-body PET, that is, examination of both the abdomen and the thorax in the same investigation despite the short half-life of ^{11}C. In a first study, eight patients with biochemically verified neuroendocrine tumors—five with suspect ACTH-producing tumors and three with EPT (2 nonfunctioning and 1 insulinoma)—underwent whole-body PET with 5-HTP in addition to MRI/CT and octreotide scintigraphy. Conventional radiology was initially considered negative in all eight cases, whereas PET could visualize tumors in six cases (three ACTH-producing tumors and all EPT). With the PET images at hand, the tumors could be identified on MRI and CT images in five cases. All six patients with positive PET examinations were operated on and the PET findings could be verified.

FDG-PET IN NEUROENDOCRINE CANCER

There is a subgroup of patients who have poorly differentiated tumors that lack somatostatin receptors and also the expression of chromogranin A in the tumors. The tumors may show the content of another marker for neuroendocrine differentiation—synaptophysin. The proliferation capacity, as evaluated by the proliferation marker Ki-67, is usually high in these tumors as compared to the more common well-differentiated neuroendocrine tumors. In this patient category, we found that PET with 5-HTP might be negative, whereas FDG-PET usually is positive and can be used for staging and therapeutic monitoring, which is in agreement with the findings of Adams *et al.*[12]

CURRENT STATUS

At present, more than 90% of neuroendocrine tumors can be visualized with PET with the tracers now available, notably HTP. PET with 5-HTP can be used to "screen" the thorax/abdomen (whole-body PET) for small primary tumors that cannot be detected by other methods including octreotide scintigraphy. In several preoperative evaluations, PET has provided crucial information to the surgeon thanks to the excellent tumor visibility, which in turn depends on the high tumor-to-background ratio and good spatial resolution. It is clear that PET with 5-HTP is the most sensitive method for detecting the extent of metastases, and is superior to octreotide scintigraphy, CT, and MRI in this respect. However, lack of availability and high cost would limit its extensive use; therefore use of PET-HTP is selective as a means in detecting neuroendocrine tumors. Especially in cases with a clinical diagnosis of neuroendocrine tumors when CT is negative or when the tumor burden is supposed to be so limited that surgery is an option, it is reasonable to use PET-HTP to exclude metastases.

PET can also be utilized to monitor functional parameters, reflecting effects of treatment on the tumors, which other methods cannot. Further, PET with FDG can be used for neuroendocrine cancers with a high proliferation index.

ADRENOCORTICAL TUMORS

As a result of the increased use of CT, MRI, and ultrasonography, accidentally detected masses at the site of the adrenals, so-called incidentalomas, are frequently revealed. Incidentalomas, reported to occur in 0.3–4% of abdominal CT investigations,[17] are in most instances benign adrenal cortical adenoma without clinical or biochemical manifestations of hormone excess. Some incidentalomas represent pheochromocytomas, metastases to the adrenal, or are of other nonadrenal origin. Presently available imaging methods are seldom capable of establishing a definite diagnosis regarding origin and potential malignancy of the lesion. Therefore, patients with incidentaloma generally must undergo more or less extensive clinical and laboratory examinations, including analyses of catecholamines and cortical hormones in urine or serum. Patients with biochemical evidence of hormone excess are generally considered for surgery. Surgery is also often advocated for tumors exceeding 3–4 cm in diameter to exclude the presence of adrenocortical carcinoma, an exceedingly rare tumor that is most often detected when it has reached conspicuous size.[18]

Our objective was to develop a PET method that would identify adrenal cortical lesions. Etomidate has been used as an anesthetic drug, but has also been documented as a potent inhibitor of 11β-hydroxylase, a key enzyme in the synthesis of cortisol and aldosterone within the adrenal cortex.[19] Metomidate, the methyl ester of etomidate, has similar properties. Preclinical studies using frozen section autoradiography showed that ^{11}C-etomidate and ^{11}C-metomidate had very high uptake in adrenal cortex and adrenal cortical tumors, but lower uptake in other examined organs, except the liver.[20] *In vivo* PET studies in monkeys demonstrated high uptake and excellent visualization of the adrenal glands. Based on better synthetic characteristics, ^{11}C-metomidate was selected as the tracer for clinical studies.

PET with this tracer was performed in 15 patients with unilateral adrenal mass > 1 cm in diameter confirmed by CT. All patients subsequently underwent surgery, except two who underwent biopsy only. The lesions were histopathologically examined and diagnosed as adrenal cortical adenoma ($n = 6$; nonfunctioning 3), adrenocortical carcinoma ($n = 2$), and nodular hyperplasia ($n = 1$). The remaining were noncortical lesions, including 1 pheochromocytoma, 1 myelolipoma, 2 adrenal cysts, and 2 metastases. All cortical lesions were easily identified because of exceedingly high uptake of ^{11}C-metomidate[21] (FIG. 3).

CONCLUSION

From this study, we conclude that ^{11}C-metomidate has the potential to be an attractive method for the characterization of adrenal masses with the ability to discriminate lesions of adrenocortical origin from noncortical lesions. In subsequent studies, the initial findings have been confirmed in a larger group of patients. In a separate study, adrenocortical cancers were investigated and also demonstrated to have very high uptake. This means that the degree of uptake per se does not discriminate adrenocortical cancers from adenomas, but irregular uptake and multiple lesions are suggestive of malignancy. ^{11}C-metomidate-PET seems, however, to be useful for staging of adrenocortical cancer as well as for post-treatment follow up.

ACKNOWLEDGMENTS

This work was supported by the Swedish Cancer Foundation, Söderberg's Foundation, and Lions Cancer Foundation.

REFERENCES

1. PEARSE, A.G.E. 1980. The APUD concept and hormone production. Clin. Endocrinol. Metab. **17:** 211–222.
2. WILLIAMS, E.D. & M. SANDLER. 1963. The classification of carcinoid tumors. Lancet **1:** 238–239.
3. THORSON, A., G. BJÖRCK, G. BJÖRKMAN, et al. 1954. Malignant carcinoid of the small intestine with metastases to the liver, valvular disease of the right side of the heart (pulmonary stenosis and tricuspid regurgitation with septal defects), peripheral vasomotor symptoms, bronchoconstriction and an unusual type of cyanosis, a clinical and pathological syndrome. Am. Heart J. **47:** 795–817.
4. NORHEIM, I., K. ÖBERG, E. THEODORSSON-NORHEIM, et al. 1987. Malignant carcinoid tumors: an analysis of 103 patients with regard to tumor localization, hormone production and survival. Ann. Surg. **206:** 115–125.

5. KRENNING, E.P., D.J. KWECKEBOOM, W.H. BAKKER, et al. 1993. Somatostatin receptor scintigraphy with [^{111}In-DTPA-D-Phe^1]- and [^{123}Tyr^3]-octreotide: the Rotterdam experience with more than 1,000 patients. Eur. J. Nucl. Med. **20:** 716–731.
6. TIENSUU JANSON, E., J.E. WESTLIN, B. ERIKSSON, et al. 1994. [^{111}In-DTPA-D-Phe^1]-Octreotide scintigraphy in patients with carcinoid tumors—the predictive value for somatostatin analogue treatment. Eur. J. Endocrinol. **131:** 575–576.
7. ERIKSSON, B. & K. ÖBERG. 1993. An update of the medical treatment of malignant endocrine pancreatic tumors. Acta Oncol. **32:** 203–208.
8. ÖBERG, K. & B. ERIKSSON. 1991. The role of interferons in the management of carcinoid tumors. Acta Oncol. **30:** 519–522.
9. ANDERSSON, T., B. ERIKSSON, P.G. LINDGREN, et al. 1990. Effects of interferon on tumor tissue content in liver metastases during interferon treatment. Cancer Res. **50:** 3413–3415.
10. IMAM, H., B. ERIKSSON, A. LUKINIUS, et al. 1997. Induction of apoptosis in neuroendocrine tumors of the digestive system during treatment with somatostatin analogs. Acta Oncol. **36:** 607–614.
11. MOERTEL, C.G., L.K. KOOLS, M.J. O'CONNELL, et al. 1991. Treatment of neuroendocrine carcinomas with combined etoposide and cisplatin. Cancer **68:** 227–232.
12. ADAMS, S., R. BAUM, T. RINK, et al. 1998. Limited value of fluorine-18 fluorodeoxyglucose positron emission tomography for the imaging of neuroendocrine tumours. Eur. J. Nucl. Med. **25:** 79–83.
13. ÖRLEFORS, H., A. SUNDIN, A. LILJA, et al. 1998. Positron emission tomography (PET) with 5-hydroxytryptophan (5-HTP) in the diagnosis and treatment follow-up of carcinoid tumors. J. Clin. Oncol. **7:** 2534–2541.
14. SUNDIN, A., B. ERIKSSON, M. BERGSTRÖM, et al. 2000. Demonstration of [^{11}C]-5-hydroxy-L-tryptophan accumulation and decarboxylation in carcinoid tumors by specific positioning labeling in positron emission tomography. Nucl. Med. Biol. **27:** 33–41.
15. BERGSTRÖM, M., L. LU, B. ERIKSSON, et al. 1996. Modulation of organ uptake of ^{11}C-labeled-5-hydroxytryptophan. Biogenic Amines **12:** 477–485.
16. AHLSTRÖM, H., B. ERIKSSON, M. BERGSTRÖM, et al. 1995. Pancreatic neuroendocrine tumors: diagnosis with PET. Radiology **195:** 333–337.
17. KLOOS, R.T., M.D. GROSS, I.R. FRANCIS, et al. 1995. Incidentally discovered adrenal masses. Endocr. Rev. **16:** 460–484.
18. GRÖNDAHL, S., B. ERIKSSON, L. HAGENÄS, et al. 1990. Steroid profile in urine: a useful tool in the diagnosis and follow up of adrenocortical carcinoma. Acta Endocrinol. **122:** 656–663.
19. WEBER, M.M., J. LANG, F. ABEDINPOUR, et al. 1993. Different inhibitory effect of etomidate and ketoconazole on the human adrenal steroid biosynthesis. Clin. Invest. **71:** 993–1038.
20. BERGSTRÖM, M., T. BONASERA, L. LU, et al. 1998. In vitro and in vivo primate evaluation of carbon-11-etomidate and carbon-11-metomidate as potential tracers for PET imaging of the adrenal cortex and its tumors. J. Nucl. Med. **39:** 982–989.
21. BERGSTRÖM, M., C. JUHLIN, T. BONASERA, et al. 2000. PET imaging of adrenal cortical tumors with the 11β-hydroxylase tracer ^{11}C-metomidate. J. Nucl. Med. **41:** 275–282.

Diagnostic Localization of Pheochromocytoma

The Coming of Age of Positron Emission Tomography

KAREL PACAK,[a] GRAEME EISENHOFER,[b] JORGE A. CARRASQUILLO,[c] CLARA C. CHEN,[c] MILLIE WHATLEY,[c] AND DAVID S. GOLDSTEIN[b]

[a]*Pediatric and Reproductive Endocrinology Branch, National Institute of Child Health and Human Development, NIH, Bethesda, Maryland 20892, USA*

[b]*Clinical Neurocardiology Section, National Institute of Neurological Disorders and Stroke, NIH, Bethesda, Maryland 20892, USA*

[c]*Nuclear Medicine Department, Clinical Center, NIH, Bethesda, Maryland 20892-1583 USA*

ABSTRACT: Pheochromocytoma is a rare but clinically important tumor of catecholamine-secreting chromaffin cells. This tumor constitutes a surgically curable cause of hypertension. Therefore, correct localization of pheochromocytoma is essential for effective management of this tumor. Several conventional and nuclear imaging modalities are currently available to localize pheochromocytoma. Computed tomography (CT) and magnetic resonance imaging (MRI) have good sensitivity but poor specificity for detecting pheochromocytoma, and nuclear imaging approaches such as ^{131}I-metaiodobenzylguanidine scintigraphy or [^{111}In]-DTPA-D-Phe-pentetreotide (Octreoscan) have limited sensitivity. However, specificity of ^{131}I-metaiodobenzylguanidine scintigraphy is very good and this means of imaging provides a method for confirming that a tumor is a pheochromocytoma and rules out metastatic disease. Recently, we introduced a new imaging method, 6-[^{18}F]fluorodopamine positron emission tomography, that can be used successfully for the detection of solitary and metastatic pheochromocytomas. Our preliminary data suggest that this method is superior to other nuclear imaging methods including metaiodobenzylguanidine and octreotide scintigraphy. In this report we provide an update regarding nuclear imaging of primary and metastatic pheochromocytoma, particularly using 6-[^{18}F]fluorodopamine positron emission tomographic scanning.

Address for correspondence: Dr. Karel Pacak, PREB, NICHD, NIH, Building 10, Room 9D42, 10 Center Drive, Bethesda, Maryland 20892. Voice: 301-402-4594; fax: 301-402-4712.
karel@mail.nih.gov

KEYWORDS: pheochromocytoma; positron emission tomography; metaiodobenzylguanidine scintigraphy; Octreoscan

CONVENTIONAL IMAGING

A variety of imaging techniques are available for localization of a pheochromocytoma. In most institutions computed tomography (CT) of the abdomen, either with or without contrast, or magnetic resonance imaging (MRI) provides initial imaging for localizing pheochromocytoma. CT or MRI localize more than 95% of pheochromocytomas but both techniques lack specificity.[1-3] MRI with or without gadolinium enhancement is superior to CT in detecting extra-adrenal tumors (almost 100% sensitivity) and familial adrenal pheochromocytoma.[2-5] Because of the characteristic T-2 weighted MRI image of pheochromocytoma, currently most institutions use this method first to exclude pheochromocytoma. MRI may also be desirable as the initial imaging procedure in children or when there is pregnancy or allergy to the contrast materials used for CT scans.

METAIODOBENZYLGUANIDINE SCINTIGRAPHY

Nuclear imaging using ^{131}I- or ^{123}I-metaiodobenzylguanidine (MIBG) scintigraphy is useful in situations where pheochromocytoma cannot be localized or for confirmation that a mass is a pheochromocytoma, or for exclusion of metastatic disease.[6-9] MIBG has almost 100% specificity but limited sensitivity. False-negative results can be particularly troublesome when ^{131}I-MIBG is used. In agreement with previously published reports, our preliminary data also show suboptimal sensitivity of ^{131}I-MIBG in the localization of metastatic pheochromocytoma. In our current series of 16 patients who presented to us with metastatic pheochromocytoma, in at least 1/3 of these patients ^{131}I-MIBG did not detect metastatic lesions detected by other imaging modalities. Undoubtedly, the use of ^{123}I-MIBG, which is clearly superior to ^{131}I-MIBG in the detection of pheochromocytoma, would be preferable. However, ^{123}I-MIBG is not FDA-approved, and its use in the United States still requires an Investigational New Drug (IND) application from the FDA. The distribution of ^{123}I-MIBG is also more problematic than of ^{131}I-MIBG since the half-life of ^{123}I is only 13 hours. Therefore, the use of ^{123}I-MIBG in the United States remains restricted to a few medical centers. Nevertheless, recently several hospitals, usually those affiliated with universities, have started using ^{123}I-MIBG, perhaps owing to the presence of private companies that provide quick and efficient distribution of this isotope directly from the manufacturer.

OCTREOSCAN

Somatostatin receptor scintigraphy using octreotide, an analogue of somatostatin, provides another method of localizing pheochromocytoma.[10–12] The conventional 6–12 mCi dose of octreotide localizes pheochromocytoma in fewer than 30% of cases.[12] In patients with a malignant pheochromocytoma, octreotide scintigraphy, however, can be useful for detection of rapidly growing tumors that have become dedifferentiated and have lost their norepinephrine transporter system (these tumors are MIBG-negative).[12] On the basis of our experience at the NIH, we do not recommend Octreoscan as a first-line imaging test for the localization of pheochromocytoma. Octreoscan should be reserved for patients in whom conventional imaging studies cannot locate the tumor, MIBG scintigraphy is negative, and 6-[^{18}F]fluorodopamine PET scanning is not available. In patients with metastatic pheochromocytoma, octreotide scintigraphy should be used in those patients in whom further treatment is planned using this compound and in whom MIBG scanning is negative.

POSITRON EMISSION TOMOGRAPHY

Several reports have described the use of positron-emitting imaging agents to visualize pheochromocytoma. Such agents include ^{18}F-fluorodeoxyglucose, ^{18}F-fluorodihydroxyphenylalanine, ^{11}C-epinephrine, and ^{11}C-hydroxyephedrine.[13–17] Imperfect sensitivity and specificity remain problems with these agents. Therefore, we sought an imaging modality that would offer both high sensitivity and specificity for diagnostic localization of this tumor. We turned our attention to 6-[^{18}F]-fluorodopamine positron emission tomographic (PET) scanning, a method initially developed at the NIH for the assessment of sympathetic nervous function.[18–21] Since catecholamine-synthesizing cells including pheochromocytoma cells posses cell membrane and intracellular vesicular transporters for catecholamines, we hypothesized that 6-[^{18}F]fluorodopamine would be a useful agent for diagnostic localization of pheochromocytoma. Furthermore, because positron-emitting agents have short half-lives, we predicted that 6-[^{18}F]fluorodopamine PET would visualize a pheochromocytoma almost immediately, in contrast to ^{131}I- or ^{123}I-metaiodobenzylguanidine scintigraphy, where an interval of up to 48–72 hours is required for optimal images.

As reviewed elsewhere,[18–21] 6-[^{18}F]fluorodopamine is transported into storage vesicles where it accumulates, enabling visualization of pheochromocytomas. The liver, pancreas, spleen, thyroid, salivary glands, nasopharyngeal mucosa, renal pelvis and cortex, and heart all concentrate 6-[^{18}F]fluorodopamine-derived radioactivity. Because of uptake or local production of metabolites of the tracer, this radioactivity does not always correlate with the density of organ sympathetic innervation. Also, the excretion of 6-[^{18}F]fluorodopamine from the gallbladder into the gut may cause some problems in terms of visualization of the right adrenal gland. However, in practice this is not a problem because of the ability to rotate the image and because 6-[^{18}F]fluorodopamine-derived radioactivity accumulates only very slowly in the gallbladder. In some cases, registration with CT or MRI is important to localize the tumor precisely.

THE USEFULNESS OF 6-[^{18}F]FLUORODOPAMINE IN THE DETECTION OF PHEOCHROMOCYTOMA

In our studies we included patients with known or suspected benign or malignant pheochromocytoma.[1,22,23] Measurements of plasma free metanephrines were used to confirm or exclude the presence of pheochromocytoma. Patients were given 1–2 mCi of 6-[^{18}F]fluorodopamine i.v. over 3 minutes. The duration of emission scanning was 8–15 minutes at each level. At least one transmission scan of 3–5 minutes duration was obtained at each level. The images were reconstructed using the MIRAGE program, which was developed by and is used routinely in the NIH Nuclear Medicine Department. The 6-[^{18}F]fluorodopamine PET scanning images were reviewed by at least two "blinded" nuclear medicine physicians and by the principal investigators.

Until now we have performed 6-[^{18}F]fluorodopamine PET in 36 patients in whom pheochromocytoma was suspected. Ten patients had solitary tumors and 12 had metastatic disease (FIG. 1). Of these patients, 13 underwent surgical removal of a tumor (10 primary and 3 metastatic tumors). All patients had elevated plasma free metanephrines, indicating the presence of pheochromocytoma, and all had positive 6-[^{18}F]fluorodopamine scans that showed primary or metastatic tumors. Three patients with positive plasma free metanephrines had negative 6-[^{18}F]fluorodopamine scans. One of these patients had progressive metastatic disease, another patient had an ACTH-producing pheochromocytoma, and the third a pheochromocytoma associated with congenital contralateral kidney agenesis. Currently tumors from these patients are under investigation; in some patients we hypothesize that a lack of norepinephrine or vesicular transporter system could cause the failure of 6-[^{18}F]fluorodopamine to localize the tumor.

Of the 14 patients with normal plasma levels of metanephrines, 12 had negative 6-[^{18}F]fluorodopamine PET scans, 1 had extra-adrenal localization of 6-[^{18}F]fluorodopamine-derived activity medial to the left kidney and in the region of the tail of the pancreas, and 1 had essentially symmetric uptake of 6-[^{18}F]fluorodopamine in the adrenal areas. Neither of the latter two patients have had surgical confirmation of these sites of 6-[^{18}F]fluorodopamine uptake.

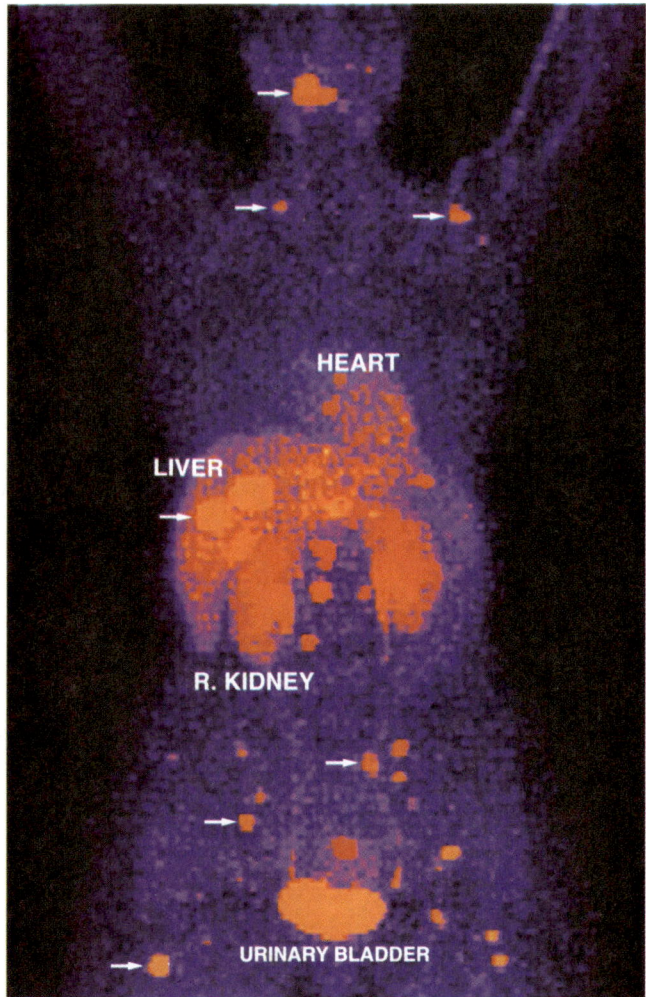

FIGURE 1. Reprojected 6-[^{18}F]fluorodopamine positron emission tomographic scan in a patient with a metastatic pheochromocytoma.

CONCLUSIONS

The present results suggest that 6-[^{18}F]fluorodopamine PET might be useful for detection and localization of pheochromocytoma. However, further studies are required to determine the extent of this usefulness, particularly in patients in whom biochemical testing is positive, but computed tomography and magnetic resonance imaging are negative. Also important is the identification of causes of positive [^{18}F]fluorodopamine PET scans in patients where biochemical tests are negative. Finally, it is important to compare results from 6-[^{18}F]fluorodopamine PET scans with other nuclear imaging methods, such as ^{131}I- or ^{123}I-metaiodobenzylguanidine scintigraphy or Octreoscan.

REFERENCES

1. PACAK, K., W.M. LINEHAN, G. EISENHOFER, et al. 2001. Recent advances in genetics, diagnosis, localization, and treatment of pheochromocytoma. Ann. Intern. Med. **134:** 315–329.
2. MAUREA, S., A. CUOCOLO, J.C. REYNOLDS, et al. 1996. Diagnostic imaging in patients with paragangliomas: computed tomography, magnetic resonance and MIBG scintigraphy comparison. Q. J. Nucl. Med. **40:** 365–371.
3. SCHMEDTJE, J.F., JR., S. SAX, J.L. POOL, et al. 1987. Localization of ectopic pheochromocytomas by magnetic resonance imaging. Am. J Med. **83:** 770–772.
4. FINK, I.J., J.W. REINIG, A.J. DWYER, et al. 1985. MR imaging of pheochromocytomas. J. Comput. Assist. Tomogr. **9:** 454–458.
5. MANGER, W.M. & R.W. GIFFORD, JR. 1993. Pheochromocytoma: current diagnosis and management. Cleveland Clin. J. Med. **60:** 365–378.
6. GOUGH, I.R., N.W. THOMPSON, B. SHAPIRO & J.C. SISSON. 1985. Limitations of 131I-MIBG scintigraphy in locating pheochromocytomas. Surgery **98:** 115–120.
7. QUINT, L.E., G.M. GLAZER, I.R. FRANCIS, et al. 1987. Pheochromocytoma and paraganglioma: comparison of MR imaging with CT and I-131 MIBG scintigraphy. Radiology. **165:** 89–93.
8. SHAPIRO, B., J.E. COPP, J.C. SISSON, et al 1985. Iodine-131 metaiodobenzylguanidine for the locating of suspected pheochromocytoma: experience in 400 cases. J. Nucl. Med. **26:** 576–585.
9. SHAPIRO, B., J.C. SISSON, B.L. SHULKIN, et al. 1995. The current status of radioiodinated metaiodobenzylguanidine therapy of neuro-endocrine tumors. Q. J. Nucl. Med. **39:** 55–57.
10. KOPF, D., A. BOCKISCH, H. STEINERT, et al. 1997. Octreotide scintigraphy and catecholamine response to an octreotide challenge in malignant phaeochromocytoma. Clin. Endocrinol. (Oxf.). **46:** 39–44.
11. KORIYAMA, N., M. KAKEI, K. YAEKURA, et al 2000. Control of catecholamine release and blood pressure with octreotide in a patient with pheochromocytoma: a case report with in vitro studies. Horm Res. **53:** 46–50.
12. VAN DER HARST, E., W.W. DE HERDER, H.A. BRUINING, et al. 2001. [(123)I]metaiodobenzylguanidine and [(111)In]octreotide uptake in benign and malignant pheochromocytomas. J. Clin. Endocrinol. Metab. **86:** 685–693.
13. SHAPIRO, B., M.D. GROSS & B. SHULKIN. 2001. Radioisotope diagnosis and therapy of malignant pheochromocytoma. Trends Endocrinol Metab. **12:** 469–475.
14. SHULKIN, B., D. WIELAND, M. SCHWAIGER, et al. 1992. PET scanning with hydroxyephedrine: a new approach to the localization of pheochromocytoma. J. Nucl. Med. **33:** 1125–1131.

15. SHULKIN, B., D. WIELAND, B. SHAPIRO & J. SISSON. 1995. PET epinephrine studies of pheochromocytoma. J. Nucl. Med. **36:** 22P–23P.
16. SHULKIN, B.L., N.W. THOMPSON, B. SHAPIRO, et al. 1999. Pheochromocytomas: imaging with 2-[Fluorine-18]fluoro-2-deoxy-D-glucose PET. Nucl Med. **212:** 35–41.
17. HOEGERLE, S., NITZSCHE, C. ALTEHOEFER, et al. 2002. Pheochromocytomas: detection with ^{18}F DOPA whole body PET: intitial results. Radiology **222:** 507–512.
18. GOLDSTEIN, D.S., P.C. CHANG, G. EISENHOFER, et al. 1990. Positron emission tomographic imaging of cardiac sympathetic innervation and function. Circulation **81:** 1606–1621.
19. GOLDSTEIN, D.S., L. CORONADO & I.J. KOPIN. 1994. 6-[Fluorine-18]fluorodopamine pharmacokinetics and dosimetry in humans. J. Nucl. Med. **35:** 964–973.
20. GOLDSTEIN, D.S., G. EISENHOFER, B.B. DUNN, et al. 1993. Positron emission tomographic imaging of cardiac sympathetic innervation using 6-[18F]fluorodopamine: initial findings in humans. J. Am. Coll. Cardiol. **22:** 1961–1971.
21. GOLDSTEIN, D.S., E. GROSSMAN, M. TAMRAT, et al. 1991. Positron emission imaging of cardiac sympathetic innervation and function using 18F-6-fluorodopamine: effects of chemical sympathectomy by 6-hydroxydopamine. J. Hypertens. **9:** 417–423.
22. PACAK, K., G. EISENHOFER, J.A. CARRASQUILLO, et al. 2001. 6-[18F]fluorodopamine positron emission tomographic (PET) scanning for diagnostic localization of pheochromocytoma. Hypertension. **38:** 6–8.
23. PACAK, K., T. FOJO, D.S. GOLDSTEIN, et al. 2001. Radiofrequency ablation: a novel approach for treatment of metastatic pheochromocytoma. J. Natl. Cancer Inst. **93:** 648–649.

Genomic Medicine

Exploring the Basis of a New Approach to Endocrine Hypertension

SALVATORE ALESCI,[a,b] GEORGE P. CHROUSOS,[a] AND KAREL PACAK[a]

[a]*Pediatric and Reproductive Endocrinology Branch, National Institute of Child Health and Human Development, National Institutes of Health, Bethesda, Maryland, 20892-1583, USA*

[b]*Sezione di Endocrinologia, Dipartimento Clinico Sperimentale di Medicina e Farmacologia, University of Messina, Messina, 98100, Italy*

ABSTRACT: Recent improvements in defining the molecular basis of disease have encouraged scientists worldwide to develop new therapeutic strategies based on engineered genes and cells. Genomic medicine has the potential to revolutionize diagnosis and therapy of a variety of human diseases, including endocrine disorders. Hypertension is the presenting feature of some of these disorders, such as congenital adrenal diseases, and adrenal and pituitary tumors. Preclinical data indicate that gene transfer to both the adrenal gland and the pituitary is not only feasible but also quite efficient. Research in this field is only in its infancy, but with the ever-increasing advances in DNA technologies, genomic therapies for endocrine hypertension may become available within the next few decades.

KEYWORDS: endocrine hypertension; gene therapy; adrenal gland; adrenal cancer; adrenocortical carcinoma; pheochromocytoma; congenital adrenal hyperplasia; hyperaldosteronism; Cushing's syndrome

INTRODUCTION: FROM GENE CLONING TO GENE-BASED MEDICINE

After the discovery of DNA in the early 1950s, scientists started dreaming of new medical treatments based on manipulations of the genome. Conse-

---

Address for correspondence: Salvatore Alesci, M.D., Pediatric and Reproductive Endocrinology Branch, National Institute of Child Health and Human Development, National Institutes of Health, Building 10, Room 9D42, 10 Center Drive MSC 1583, Bethesda, MD 20892-1583. Voice: 301-496-0610; fax: 301-402-7572.

alescis@mail.nih.gov

quently, over the last decades, significant efforts have been made to analyze nucleic acid structure and function in health and disease. The explosion of recombinant DNA and gene cloning technologies have enabled researchers to explore the potential of novel therapeutic strategies based on engineered genes and cells, making an old dream come true.

Gene therapy (GT) implies introduction of foreign genes (transgenes) into patients' cells to change the natural course of their disease by either correcting genetic defects or overexpressing therapeutically useful molecules. Originally applied to the treatment of monogenic diseases, today GT has been proposed as a powerful means of treating many polygenic disorders, including endocrine diseases and cancers.

Since the first clinical trial of GT in 1990,[1] more than 400 clinical protocols have been approved worldwide, and more than 5000 patients have been treated.[2] However, despite few reports of successful therapeutic responses in patients treated by GT,[3,4] the current clinical experience suggests inadequate efficacy and safety.[5] Nevertheless, with the recent advances in "genomic" and "proteomic" technologies, gene- and cell-based medicine is likely to become available to the general public within the next decades.

GENE DELIVERY SYSTEMS: CHASING THE IDEAL VECTOR

Gene delivery to somatic cells (transduction) can take place either *ex vivo* or *in vivo*. In the *ex vivo* approach, cells removed from the patient are engineered *in vitro*, followed by reimplantantion into the host. This method has the advantage of a more efficient gene transfer, because engineered cells can be propagated and exposed to large amounts of the vector for prolonged periods of time. However, it also suffers from patient-specificity, applicability to only transplantable cell types (i.e., lymphocytes, bone marrow cells, stem cells, hepatocytes, skin fibroblasts), and priced manufacturing.

The *in vivo* approach involves direct administration of the transgene construct to the patient, and it is therefore less costly, but also less efficient.

The ideal GT vector should satisfy all of the following requirements: (1) easy production at high titers; (2) proficient delivery of transgenes of any size to both mitotic and postmitotic cells; (3) site-specific integration into the host genome; (4) prolonged and regulated transgene expression; (5) safety. Unfortunately, not all these properties are simultaneously present in any of the currently available vectors. At present, there are five major categories of gene-delivery systems: viral, synthetic, hybrid viral-synthetic, physical, and engineered stem cells. Properties of the most commonly used gene vectors are summarized in TABLE 1.

TABLE 1. Comparative oveview of the properties of the most common gene delivery systems

Delivery system	Insert capacity	Titer (cfu[a]/ml)	Target cells	Transduction efficiency		Length of gene expression	Safety issues
				in vitro	in vivo		
Adenovirus	7–35 kb	10^8–10^{11}	mitotic; post-mitotic	Very high	Very high	Short	Immunogenicity
Retrovirus	8 kb	10^6–10^9	mitotic	High	Low	Long	Insertional mutagenesis
Lentivirus	8 kb	10^9–10^{10}	mitotic; post-mitotic	High	High	Long	HIV origins
Adeno-associated virus	4.5 kb	10^6–10^9	mitotic; post-mitotic	High	High	Very long	Little clinical experience
Naked DNA	>20 kb	N/A	mitotic; post-mitotic	Very low	Very low	Very short	Good safety profile
DNA–lipid complexes	No size limit	N/A	mitotic; post-mitotic	High	Very low	Very short	Good safety profile
DNA–polymers complexes	No size limit	N/A	mitotic; post-mitotic	High	Low	Very short	Good safety profile
Physical methods	No size limit	N/A	mitotic; post-mitotic	Moderate	Low	Very short	Little clinical experience

[a]colony-forming units.

Recombinant Viral Vectors

Recombinant viral vectors are derived from viruses by replacing genes involved in the viral pathogenesis with the transgene of interest. The most frequently used viral vectors in clinical trials are adenoviruses (AVs) and retroviruses (RVs), while lentiviruses (LVs)[6] and adeno-associated viruses (AAVs)[7] are in preclinical or early clinical testing.

Human AVs are nonenveloped viruses causing benign infections in several organs, including upper respiratory tract, eye, urinary bladder, gastrointestinal tract, and liver. The adenoviral genome consists of a single double-stranded linear DNA molecule (36 kb). It includes early (*E1A, E1B, E2, E3, and E4*), delayed (*IX and IVa2*), and late (*L1–L5*) transcriptional units, expressed at different times during the viral replicative cycle. It also contains a *cis*-acting packaging signal (Ψ) and two inverted terminal repeats (ITRs) to control the host transcriptional machinery[8] (FIG. 1A). Replication-deficient

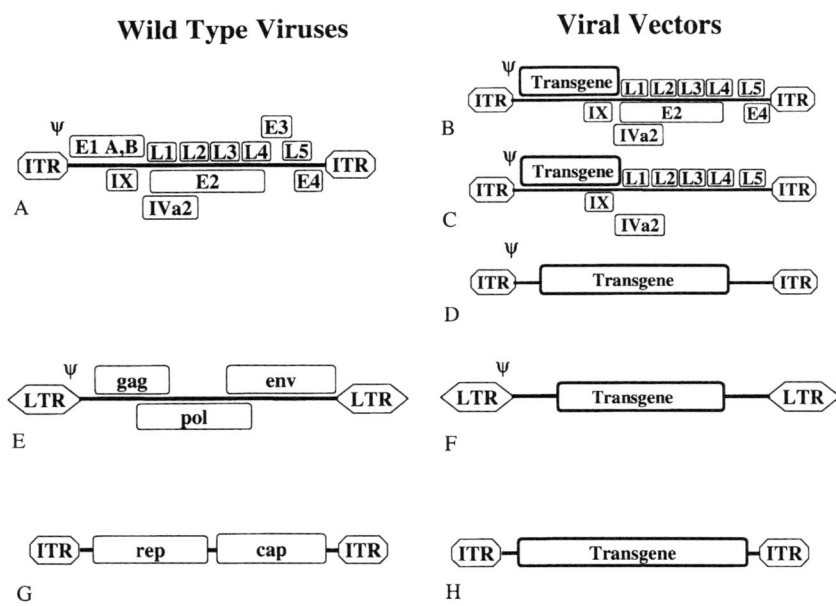

FIGURE 1. Genomic organization of wild-type viruses (*left*) versus recombinant viral vectors for gene therapy (*right*) derived from them: (**A**) wild-type adenovirus; (**B**) first-generation E1/E3 deleted adenoviral vector; (**C**) second-generation E1/E2/E3/E4 deleted adenoviral vector; (**D**) "gutless" adenoviral vector; (**E**) wild-type retrovirus; (**F**) retroviral vector; (**G**) wild-type adeno-associated virus; (**H**) adeno-associated viral vector.

adenoviral vectors, mainly derived from AVs serotypes 5, 2, 7, and 4, can be produced at high titers (as high as 10^{11} colony-forming units [cfu] per mL) using different packaging cell lines.[9] These vectors attain transient but effective transgene expression in both dividing and nondividing cells. However, they do not integrate into the host genome, usually remaining episomal.[10] First-generation AV vectors, deleted in the *E1* and *E3* genes (FIG. 1B), are still able to express most of the viral genes. Their products, once exposed on the surface of the host cells, elicit a strong immune response, a process that leads to elimination of the host's transduced cells, therefore annulling the transgene expression.[11] Second-generation adenoviral vectors are derived from the first generation by further deletion of the E2 and/or E4 regions (FIG. 1C), while the most recent "gutless" vectors have all the viral genome deleted except for the Ψ and ITR sequences (FIG. 1D). These adenoviral vectors are less immunogenic and have higher cloning capacity.[12]

Because AVs are a common cause of mild respiratory infections in humans, most of the patients undergoing adenoviral-based GT already have neutralizing antiviral antibodies circulating in their blood, another element that may limit the efficacy of the treatment. Use of nonhuman adenoviral vectors can overcome this limitation only in part. In fact, a neutralizing immune response will still follow the first GT application, interfering with repeated dosing. The strong immune response associated with the use of AV vectors may be a problem for corrective gene therapy of hereditary disorders, which often require life-long transgene expression. On the other hand, this may be beneficial for cancer gene therapy, especially if combined with the lytic action of replicating AVs. Indeed, viral oncolysis, which uses adenoviral mutants (such as dl1520 or ONYX-015) preferentially targeting cancer cells to deliver therapeutic molecules to the tumor, has shown promising results.[13,14]

RVs are enveloped RNA viruses. Their single-stranded genome (7–10 kb) include three genes (*env, gag, pol*) encoding structural viral proteins and viral enzymes, plus a *cis*-acting Ψ and long terminal repeats (LTRs) sequences[15] (FIG. 1E). Recombinant retroviral vectors are deleted in their entire genome except for Ψ and LTRs (FIG. 1F). The missing viral genes are provided in *trans* by packaging cell lines.[16] Unlike AVs, RVs enter the host cell nucleus only at mitosis, thus they can transduce only proliferating cells. Another difference RVs have with AVs is the ability to integrate into the target-cell chromosome, a process that *in vitro* usually leads to a more prolonged transgene expression. Unfortunately, the length of the expression is shorter *in vivo*, partially because of a rapid inactivation by the complement system. Major limitations in the use of these vectors also include relatively low titers (10^6–10^9 cfu per mL); insert-size capacity (8 kb); potential risk of oncogene activation or tumor suppressor gene inactivation by insertional mutagenesis; generation of replication-competent retroviral vectors through recombination with RVs resident in the human genome in cryptic form.[17]

LVs are complex retroviruses that have acquired the ability to infect postmitotic cells, overcoming a major limitation of other RVs.[18,19] The first LV vectors were derived from the human immunodeficiency virus (HIV).[20] To minimize the risk of generating wild-type infectious HIV virions in packaging cells, transmittable to the patient at the time of delivery, researchers have tried to delete as many viral accessory genes as possible, without affecting the ability of the virus to infect nondividing cells.[21] In addition, the use of nonhuman LVs, such as simian immunodeficiency virus, feline immunodeficiency virus, equine infectious anemia virus, and ovine maedi/visna virus, may also decrease the chances of generating replication-competent HIV vectors.[22] There are currently no clinical studies using lentiviral vectors.

AAVs are nonpathogenic viruses, commonly found in the human respiratory and gastrointestinal systems. Their single-stranded DNA contains a structural gene (*cap*), a regulatory gene (*rep*), and two small ITRs[23] (FIG. 1G). In order to replicate, AAVs require extra genes, which are provided by a "helper virus," usually an AV or herpes simplex virus (HSV).[24] In the absence of a helper virus, AAVs naturally integrate into a specific region of the human chromosome 19, the AAVS1 site,[25] and remain latent. AAV vectors are produced by complete or partial deletion of the *rep* and *cap* genes (FIG. 2H) and cotransfection of AV-infected cells, followed by heat inactivation to remove any residual helper virus. In fact, while AVs are heat labile, AAVs are heat stable.[24] AAVs, which have a broad cell tropism, give stable and prolonged transgene expression both *in vitro* and *in vivo*.[26–28] However, recombinant AAVs integrate into the host genome less efficiently and more randomly than wild-type viruses. Some of them remain episomal, but may persist in the host cells for long periods of time.[29] According to a study, about 30% of adult humans have preexisting antibodies against AAV serotype 2.[30] However, clinical data on the immunogenicity of AAV vectors are sparse. Despite some improvements, the main disadvantage of AAV vectors remains their manufacturing, which includes problems of low titer, AV contamination, and costly purification.[31] Another problem is the small insert size, which is limited to about 4.5 kb.

Other viruses currently tested as vectors for GT include HSVs,[32] poxviruses,[33] Sindbis and Semliki Forest alphaviruses,[34] the Sendai virus,[35] and the Epstein–Barr virus.[36] The most promising among them are HSVs, which, because of the size of their genome (150 kb), can accommodate very large transgenes. On the other hand, the complexity of their genome, containing more than 80 genes, makes the engineering of HSV vectors difficult.[32] Further limitation to their use may be the risk of neurologic complications.

Finally, some researchers are developing hybrid viral vectors, incorporating components of different viruses, such as chimeric AVs/RVs[37] and AVs/AAVs.[38]

Synthetic Vectors

Synthetic vectors include naked DNA and DNA complexes with liposomes or polymers. Naked DNA has produced efficient transgene expression after local injection in the skin[39] and muscle.[40] Other tissues, such as thyroid gland,[41] liver,[42] and endothelium,[43] have been transduced using naked DNA, but with lower efficiency. The mechanism of transfection by naked DNA is still unclear. After a rapid internalization into the cell, DNA translocates to the nucleus, where it remains episomal for extended periods of time.[44] The most promising applications of this approach include the development of genomic vaccines.[45] The main disadvantages of this method are low gene-delivery efficiency and brief expression in most tissues, especially *ex vivo*.

Liposomes have been used for years to deliver therapeutic compounds to cells.[46] Similarly, liposomes and polymers have been developed to deliver nucleic acids into the cells. DNA binds to cationic lipids through its negatively charged phosphate groups. The DNA–liposome complexes have a net positive surface charge, and are therefore able to bind sialic acid groups expressed on the plasmamembrane of target cells.[47] Following uptake, the DNA is somehow released from the complexes into the cytosol and remains extrachromosomal. Being free of protein, liposome complexes are less immunogenic than other GT systems: for this reason, they are usually considered safe. However, toxic reactions have been documented both *in vitro*[48] and *in vivo*.[49] The main disadvantages of this gene delivery method are poor and nonspecific targeting, rapid clearance from the blood, and low efficiency *in vivo*.

Cationic polymers used to complex DNA include polylysine and polyethyleneimine.[50] DNA–polymer complexes are often too large to be efficiently taken up by the cell. In addition, following uptake, they may be trapped into endosome vesicles, requiring administration of exogenous disrupting agents to achieve a significant transfection level. Such agents, though, may be used *in vitro* but not *in vivo*. There are currently no clinical studies employing DNA–polymer complexes.

Hybrid Viral–Synthetic Vectors

To combine the efficient transgene expression of viral-mediated DNA transfer with the low toxicity and good safety profile of synthetic GT vectors, researchers are now developing hybrid viral–synthetic vectors, where synthetic components, such as cationic lipids, are merged with viral proteins. Research in this field is very promising.[51]

Physical Methods

DNA can be physically transferred to target cells through needle-free injectors or electric fields. Needle-free devices use high-pressure gas ("gene-gun") or liquid ("jetgun") to deliver DNA-coated gold particles directly into the cell cytoplasm or interstitial space.[52,53] Both methods give moderate but transient transduction in the skin and muscle *in vivo* and, like naked DNA, are a promising tool for the development of genetic vaccines.[54] Electroporation, the delivery of exogenous DNA into cells through electric fields, has been tested on mice tumors.[55] Other experimental physical strategies for transgene delivery include catheter-mediated gene transfer,[56] and injection of biodegradable DNA-coated microspheres.[57]

Engineered Stem Cells

The use of stem cells, genetically engineered *ex vivo* and then reintroduced into the patient, is one of the newest and most promising gene delivery strategies. Human stem cells have recently generated great interest in both the lay and biomedical communities. The main advantage of using stem cells for GT could be the ability to continually replenish pools of differentiated cells, without the need for frequent readministration, which makes them a very appealing transfer vehicle for corrective GT. Human hematopoietic, mesenchymal, neuronal, and embryonic stem cells have been well characterized and are currently being tested for therapeutic angiogenesis, Parkinson's disease, bone marrow transplantation, and AIDS.[58,59]

GENE DELIVERY INTO ENDOCRINE TISSUES: NEW PERSPECTIVES FOR THE TREATMENT OF ENDOCRINE CAUSES OF HYPERTENSION

The application of DNA technology in endocrinology has led to a better understanding of the molecular basis of inherited and acquired endocrine diseases. Nevertheless, endocrine GT is still at a very early stage and only a few research groups, including ours, have started investigating the feasibility, effectiveness, and safety of gene transfer to endocrine cells.

One of the most appealing applications of genomic medicine in endocrinology could be the treatment of endocrine hypertension. In fact, hypertension is not only a debilitating disease, with an enormous socioeconomic and emotional impact, but also a common manifestation of a variety of endocrine disorders. These include endocrine tumors, which often respond poorly to current treatments. These tumors would greatly benefit from alternative therapies, including GT.

Gene Delivery into the Adrenal Gland

Endocrine hypertension is often identified with adrenal hypertension, which may result from excessive production of glucocorticoids, mineralocorticoids, or catecholamines. Glucocorticoid and mineralocorticoid excess can be caused by adrenocortical tumors or congenital adrenal disorders.

Adrenocortical carcinomas are highly malignant tumors, often presenting with features of adrenocortical hyperactivity, including Cushing's syndrome and virilization.[60] Although surgical resection is currently the only curative option, as many as 70% of the patients already have metastatic lesions at the time the diagnosis is made, precluding any curative resection. Mitotane is often used alone or in combination with other chemotherapeutic agents, but it does not significantly improve the life expectancy of most patients.[61]

Aldosterone-secreting adrenal adenomas are the most common cause of primary hyperaldosteronism associated with mineralocorticoid hypertension (Conn's syndrome). These benign tumors produce aldosterone independently of renin and may be found in up to 10% of patients with high blood pressure. The surgical outcome in patients with aldosterone-secreting adenomas depends on several factors, including age, duration of hypertension, presence of renal impairment, and prior response to medical treatment. Laparoscopic adrenalectomy is the treatment of choice. However, many aldosterone-secreting adenomas are smaller than 1 cm in diameter, which is below the detection limit of computerized tomography scanning and require a more invasive diagnostic procedure, such as adrenal venous sampling.[62] A less common cause of primary hyperaldosteronism are aldosterone-producing carcinomas, often widely metastatic at the time of diagnosis.[63]

Rare genetic errors of adrenal steroid metabolism can also present with hypertension. Deficiency of 17α- and 11β-hydroxylases cause inability to synthesize cortisol, resulting in excessive production of deoxycorticosterone, which acts as a mineralocorticoid. 11β-hydroxysteroid dehydrogenase deficiency causes decreased peripheral conversion of cortisol to cortisone. The delayed removal of the glucocorticoid from strategic receptors unmasks potential sites for mineralocorticoid agonism, especially in the kidney.[64] As in many genetic diseases, the current treatment of congenital adrenal enzymopathies is aimed at improving symptoms rather than at correcting the causative defects.

Pheochromocytomas are rare tumors of the adrenal medulla associated with persistently elevated blood pressure and/or paroxysms of hypertension, caused by excessive release of norepinephrine and/or epinephrine. About 10% of these neuroendocrine tumors are hereditary, most often associated with multiple endocrine neoplasia type 2 (MEN 2), von Hippel-Lindau disease, and neurofibromatosis type 1.[65] Although 90% of pheochromocytomas are benign, 10% are malignant, highly metastatic, and refractory to any current treatment.[66]

Some evidence suggests that the adrenal gland is a major target for viral vectors used in GT. In fact, persistent transgene expression within the adrenal gland has incidentally been reported in animal studies using recombinant viral vectors for fetal GT.[67–69] More interestingly, a single intra-adrenal injection of an adenoviral vector encoding the cytochrome P450 21-hydroxylase gene, transiently compensated endocrine and histologic alterations in a mouse model of 21-hydroxylase deficiency, a congenital adrenal disease.[70] Transduction of bovine adrenal zona glomerulosa cells with a recombinant adenovirus encoding the endothelial nitric oxide synthetase was associated with decreased aldosterone synthesis by transduced cells.[71] In addition, AV-mediated transfer of a suicide gene has been tested successfully in mouse and human adrenocortical cell lines.[72]

Based on these few pieces of evidence, we have started investigating the effect of *in vitro* transduction by recombinant viral vectors on the morphology and physiology of adrenal cells. We recently reported extremely high levels of transgene expression in bovine adrenal cortical cells transduced by an E1/E3-deleted AV vector expressing a modified form of the *Aequorea victoria* green fluorescent protein (GFP), which was documented by fluorescence microscopy (FIG. 2). Cell transduction with this vector was accompanied by mitochondrial and nuclear alterations, increased cell proliferation, increased basal steroidogenesis, and suppressed ACTH-stimulated steroidogenesis. Interestingly, use of two different AV mutants, partially or totally deleted in the E4 region, did not alter adrenocortical cell steroid secretion.[73]

We concluded that, given the very efficient AV-mediated transgene expression in adrenocortical cells transduced *in vitro*, AV vectors may be suitable for GT of adrenal disorders, as long as they are appropriately engineered to not alter the adrenal physiology.[73] Our results, combined with the ability of transplanted bovine and human adrenocortical cells to reconstitute fully functional adrenal tissue,[74] suggest that the adrenal gland may be a good candidate for *ex vivo* GT. Based on this evidence, we are currently extending our studies to other GT vectors and adrenal cell models, including chromaffin and pheochromocytoma cells, in order to collect the largest amount of information from these experimental studies before, eventually, going to clinical trials.

Gene Delivery into the Pituitary Gland

Acromegaly caused by growth hormone (GH)-secreting somatotroph tumors, and Cushing's disease caused by corticotroph tumors secreting ACTH and other proopiomelanocortin precursor peptides, are rare, but both associated with significant hypertension. Despite recent advances, current treatments for pituitary tumors are often unsatisfactory. In acromegaly, surgery is frequently useful in reducing tumor mass and the associated symptoms. However, it does not completely cure the GH excess. On the other hand, medical therapy does not significantly affect tumor size, though it is more effective in treating the endocrine excess, but with potentially long-term side effects. Finally, irradiation is proven to reduce the risk of postoperative tumor progression, although panhypopituitarism and impaired memory can be the price to

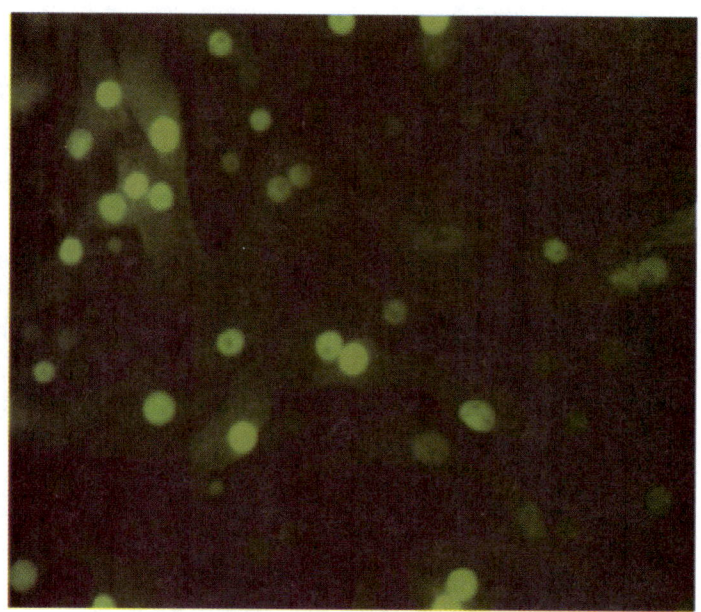

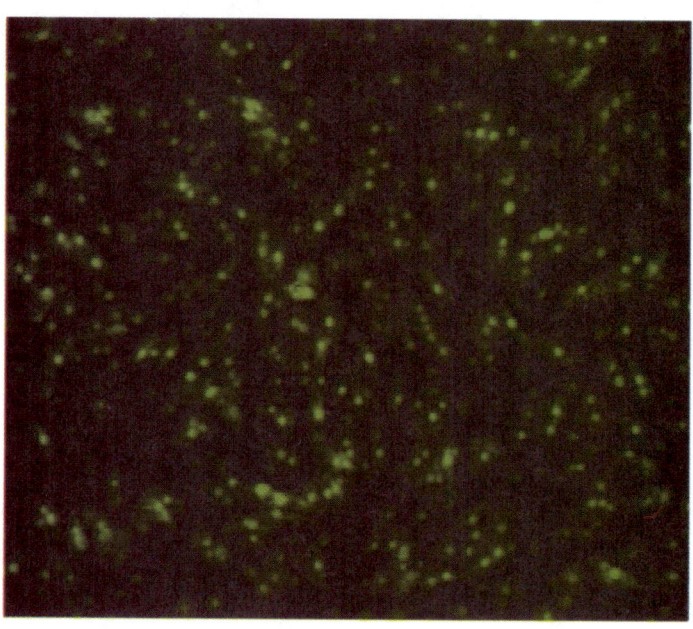

FIGURE 2. Fluorescence microscopy photographs of bovine adrenal cortical cells transduced by an E1/E3 deleted adenoviral vector engineered to express an enhanced green fluorescent protein. Twenty-four hours after transduction, high levels of transgene expression were observed in 90–100% of the cells. *Left panel*: 10× magnification; *right panel*: 40× magnification.

pay for this beneficial effect.[75] Therefore, alternative therapeutic strategies, including GT, may be desirable.[76]

Interestingly, recombinant adenoviral vectors have been successfully used for gene transfer into the anterior pituitary gland both *in vitro*[77–79] and *in vivo*.[80] Adenoviral vectors have been employed to transduce pituitary adenoma cell lines and animal models with the HSV thymidine kinase product.[81] Cell-type specific adenoviral-mediated transgene expression was achieved in the pituitary gland using the GH gene promoter.[77,78] Recombinant retroviruses were tested on the AtT20 pituitary cell line,[82,83] but the efficiency of transduction was low. Recombinant temperature-sensitive HSV type 1 vectors have also been employed for gene transfer into pituitary tumors and normal anterior pituitary cells.[84]

CONCLUSION

Hypertension is a feature of a number of endocrine disorders, including adrenal and pituitary diseases. Experimental studies on gene targeting to these endocrine tissues are promising, suggesting that genomic medicine might be applicable to the diagnosis and treatment of endocrine hypertension. However, research in this field is only in its early phase and identification of suitable genes and appropriate delivery systems will require time and effort. Testing of the efficacy and safety of genomic therapies in preclinical models of disease is an essential step toward their successful clinical application.

ACKNOWLEDGMENTS

We thank Shiromi Perera for her editorial assistance and Keith Zachman for his technical assistance. This work is part of a Ph.D. program from the University of Messina, Italy, in collaboration with the Pediatric and Reproductive Endocrinology Branch at the National Institute of Child Health and Human Development, National Institutes of Health, Bethesda, Maryland.

REFERENCES

1. BLAESE, R.M. *et al.* 1995. T lymphocyte-directed gene therapy for ADA-SCID: initial trial results after 4 years. Science **270:** 475–480.
2. ANONYMOUS. 1999. Gene transfer and therapy clinical trials—update. Part I: Countries, diseases, clinical trial phases, routes of administration. J. Gene Med. **1:** 71–73.
3. CAVAZZANA-CALVO, M. *et al.* 2000. Gene therapy of human severe combined immunodeficiency (SCID)-X1 disease. Science **288:** 669–672.

4. KAY, M.A. *et al.* 2000. Evidence for gene transfer and expression of factor IX in haemophilia B patients treated with an AAV vector. Nat. Genet. **24:** 257–261.
5. VERMA, I.M. & N. SOMIA. 1997. Gene therapy—promises, problems and prospects. Nature **389:** 239–242.
6. AMADO, R.G. & I.S. CHEN. 1999. Lentiviral vectors—the promise of gene therapy within reach? Science **285:** 674–676.
7. MONAHAN, P.E. & R.J. SAMULSKI. 2000. AAV vectors: is clinical success on the horizon? Gene Ther. **7:** 24–30.
8. SHENK, T. 1996. Adenoviridae: the viruses and their replication. *In* Fundamental Virology. B.N. Fields, Ed.: 979–1016. Lippincot-Raven. Philadelphia, PA.
9. GRAHAM, F. & L. PREVEC. 1991. Manipulation of adenovirus vectors. *In* Methods in Molecular Biology. Gene Transfer and Expression Techniques, Vol. 7. E.M.J. Walker, Ed.: 109–128. Humana Press. Clifton, NJ.
10. HARUI, A. *et al.* 1999. Frequency and stability of chromosomal integration of adenovirus vectors. J. Virol. **73:** 6141–6146.
11. NEWMAN, K.D. *et al.* 1995. Adenovirus-mediated gene transfer into normal rabbit arteries results in prolonged vascular cell activation, inflammation, and neointimal hyperplasia. J. Clin. Invest. **96:** 2955–2965.
12. WILSON, J.M. 1996. Adenoviruses as gene-delivery vehicles. N. Engl. J. Med. **334:** 1185–1187.
13. HERMISTON, T. 2000. Gene delivery from replication-selective viruses: arming guided missiles in the war against cancer. J. Clin. Invest. **105:** 1169–1172.
14. ALEMANY, R., C. BALAGUE & D.T. CURIEL. 2000. Replicative adenoviruses for cancer therapy. Nat. Biotechnol. **18:** 723–727.
15. COFFIN, J. 1996. Retroviridae: the viruses and their classification. *In* Fileds Virology. B.N. Fields, Ed.: 1767–1848. Lippincot-Raven. Philadelphia, PA.
16. MILLER, A. 1997. Development and application of retroviral vectors. *In* Retroviruses. J.M Coffin and H.E. Varmus, Eds.: 437–473. Cold Spring Harbor Laboratory Press. Plainview, NY.
17. NABEL, E.G. & G.J. NABEL. 1994. Complex models for the study of gene function in cardiovascular biology. Annu. Rev. Physiol. **56:** 741–761.
18. LEWIS, P., M. HENSEL & M. EMERMAN. 1992. Human immunodeficiency virus infection of cells arrested in the cell cycle. EMBO J. **11:** 3053–3058.
19. NALDINI, L. *et al.* 1996. *In vivo* gene delivery and stable transduction of nondividing cells by a lentiviral vector. Science **272:** 263–267.
20. POESCHLA, E., P. CORBEAU & F. WONG-STAAL. 1996. Development of HIV vectors for anti-HIV gene therapy. Proc. Natl. Acad Sci USA **93:** 11395–11399.
21. ZUFFEREY, R. *et al.* 1997. Multiply attenuated lentiviral vector achieves efficient gene delivery *in vivo*. Nat. Biotechnol. **15:** 871–875.
22. MIYOSHI, H. *et al.* 1998. Development of a self-inactivating lentivirus vector. J. Virol. **72:** 8150–8157.
23. BERNS, K. 1996. Parvoviridae: the viruses and their replication. *In* Fields Virology. B.N. Fields, Ed.: 2173–2197. Lippincot-Raven. Philadelphia, PA.
24. CARTER, B.J. 1992. Adeno-associated virus vectors. Curr. Opin. Biotechnol. **3:** 533–539.
25. KOTIN, R.M., R.M. LINDEN & K.I. BERNS. 1992. Characterization of a preferred site on human chromosome 19q for integration of adeno-associated virus DNA by non-homologous recombination. EMBO J. **11:** 5071–5078.

26. DONAHUE, B.A. *et al.* 1999. Selective uptake and sustained expression of AAV vectors following subcutaneous delivery. J. Gene Med. **1:** 31–42.
27. CONRAD, C.K. *et al.* 1996. Safety of single-dose administration of an adeno-associated virus (AAV)-CFTR vector in the primate lung. Gene Ther. **3:** 658–668.
28. WAGNER, J.A. *et al.* 1998. Efficient and persistent gene transfer of AAV-CFTR in maxillary sinus. Lancet **351:** 1702–1703.
29. MALIK, P. *et al.* 1997. Recombinant adeno-associated virus mediates a high level of gene transfer but less efficient integration in the K562 human hematopoietic cell line. J. Virol. **71:** 1776–1783.
30. CHIRMULE, N. *et al.* 1999. Immune responses to adenovirus and adeno-associated virus in humans. Gene Ther. **6:** 1574–1583.
31. FERRARI, F.K. *et al.* 1997. New developments in the generation of Ad-free, high-titer rAAV gene therapy vectors. Nat. Med. **3:** 1295–1297.
32. KRISKY, D.M. *et al.* 1998. Deletion of multiple immediate-early genes from herpes simplex virus reduces cytotoxicity and permits long-term gene expression in neurons. Gene Ther. **5:** 1593–1603.
33. SANDA, M.G. *et al.* 1999. Recombinant vaccinia-PSA (PROSTVAC) can induce a prostate-specific immune response in androgen-modulated human prostate cancer. Urology **53:** 260–266.
34. POLO, J.M. *et al.* 1999. Stable alphavirus packaging cell lines for Sindbis virus and Semliki Forest virus-derived vectors. Proc. Natl. Acad. Sci. USA **96:** 4598–4603.
35. NAKANISHI, M. *et al.* 1999. Gene delivery systems using the Sendai virus. Mol. Membr. Biol. **16:** 123–127.
36. ROBERTSON, E.S., T. OOKA & E.D. KIEFF. 1996. Epstein-Barr virus vectors for gene delivery to B lymphocytes. Proc. Natl. Acad. Sci. USA **93:** 11334–11340.
37. DUISIT, G. *et al.* 1999. Functional characterization of adenoviral/retroviral chimeric vectors and their use for efficient screening of retroviral producer cell lines. Hum. Gene Ther. **10:** 189–200.
38. FISHER, K.J. *et al.* 1996. A novel adenovirus-adeno-associated virus hybrid vector that displays efficient rescue and delivery of the AAV genome. Hum. Gene Ther. **7:** 2079–2087.
39. HENGGE, U.R. *et al.* 1995. Cytokine gene expression in epidermis with biological effects following injection of naked DNA. Nat. Genet. **10:** 161–166.
40. WOLFF, J.A. *et al.* 1990. Direct gene transfer into mouse muscle *in vivo*. Science **247:** 1465–1468.
41. SIKES, M.L. *et al.* 1994. *In vivo* gene transfer into rabbit thyroid follicular cells by direct DNA injection. Hum. Gene Ther. **5:** 837–844.
42. Malone, R.W. *et al.* 1994. Dexamethasone enhancement of gene expression after direct hepatic DNA injection. J. Biol. Chem. **269:** 29903–29907.
43. RIESSEN, R. *et al.* 1993. Arterial gene transfer using pure DNA applied directly to a hydrogel-coated angioplasty balloon. Hum. Gene Ther. **4:** 749–758.
44. WOLFF, J.A. *et al.* 1992. Long-term persistence of plasmid DNA and foreign gene expression in mouse muscle. Hum. Mol. Genet. **1:** 363–369.
45. WANG, R. *et al.* 1998. Induction of antigen-specific cytotoxic T lymphocytes in humans by a malaria DNA vaccine. Science **282:** 476–480.
46. HEATH, T.D., N.G. LOPEZ & D. PAPAHADJOPOULOS. 1985. The effects of liposome size and surface charge on liposome-mediated delivery of methotrexate-gamma-aspartate to cells *in vitro*. Biochim. Biophys. Acta **820:** 74–84.

47. FELGNER, J.H. *et al.* 1994. Enhanced gene delivery and mechanism studies with a novel series of cationic lipid formulations. J. Biol. Chem. **269:** 2550–2561.
48. FELGNER, P.L. *et al.* 1987. Lipofection: a highly efficient, lipid-mediated DNA-transfection procedure. Proc. Natl. Acad. Sci. USA **84:** 7413–7417.
49. LI, S. & L. HUANG. 2000. Nonviral gene therapy: promises and challenges. Gene Ther. **7:** 31–34.
50. BOUSSIF, O., M.A. ZANTA & J.P. BEHR. 1996. Optimized galenics improve *in vitro* gene transfer with cationic molecules up to 1000-fold. Gene Ther. **3:** 1074–1080.
51. KANEDA, Y. 1999. Development of a novel fusogenic viral liposome system (HVJ-liposomes) and its applications to the treatment of acquired diseases. Mol. Membr. Biol. **16:** 119–122.
52. CONDON, C. *et al.* 1996. DNA-based immunization by *in vivo* transfection of dendritic cells. Nat. Med. **2:** 1122–1128.
53. MATHEI, C., P. VAN DAMME & A. MEHEUS. 1997. Hepatitis B vaccine administration: comparison between jet-gun and syringe and needle. Vaccine **15:** 402–404.
54. TACKET, C.O. *et al.* 1999. Phase 1 safety and immune response studies of a DNA vaccine encoding hepatitis B surface antigen delivered by a gene delivery device. Vaccine **17:** 2826–2829.
55. NISHI, T. *et al.* 1997. Treatment of cancer using pulsed electric field in combination with chemotherapeutic agents or genes. Hum. Cell **10:** 81–86.
56. BOEKSTEGERS, P. *et al.* 2000. Myocardial gene transfer by selective pressure-regulated retroinfusion of coronary veins. Gene Ther. **7:** 232–240.
57. BANAI, S. *et al.* 1994. Angiogenic-induced enhancement of collateral blood flow to ischemic myocardium by vascular endothelial growth factor in dogs. Circulation **89:** 2183–2189.
58. ASAHARA, T., C. KALKA & J.M. ISNER. 2000. Stem cell therapy and gene transfer for regeneration. Gene Ther. **7:** 451–457.
59. GAGE, F.H. 1998. Cell therapy. Nature **392:** 18–24.
60. KASPERLIK-ZALUSKA, A.A. *et al.* 1995. Adrenocortical carcinoma. A clinical study and treatment results of 52 patients. Cancer **75:** 2587–2591.
61. DEMEURE, M.J. & L.B. SOMBERG. 1998. Functioning and nonfunctioning adrenocortical carcinoma: clinical presentation and therapeutic strategies. Surg. Oncol. Clin. N. Am. **7:** 791–805.
62. LO, C.Y. *et al.* 1996. Primary aldosteronism. Results of surgical treatment. Ann. Surg. **224:** 125–130.
63. MELBY, J.C. 1989. Clinical review 1: endocrine hypertension. J. Clin. Endocrinol. Metab. **69:** 697–703.
64. ULICK, S. & M.D. CHU. 1982. Hypersecretion of a new corticosteroid, 18-hydroxycortisol in two types of adrenocortical hypertension. Clin. Exp. Hypertens. A **4:** 1771–1777.
65. KOCH, C.A. *et al.* 2001. Genetic aspects of pheochromocytoma. Endocr. Regul. **35:** 43–52.
66. PACAK, K. *et al.* 2001. Recent advances in genetics, diagnosis, localization, and treatment of pheochromocytoma. Ann. Intern. Med. **134:** 315–329.
67. SCHACHTNER, S. *et al.* 1999. Temporally regulated expression patterns following in utero adenovirus-mediated gene transfer. Gene Ther. **6:** 1249–1257.
68. SENOO, M. *et al.* 2000. Adenovirus-mediated in utero gene transfer in mice and guinea pigs: tissue distribution of recombinant adenovirus determined by

quantitative TaqMan-polymerase chain reaction assay. Mol. Genet. Metab. **69:** 269–276.
69. YANG, E.Y. *et al.* 1999. BAPS Prize—1997. Fetal gene therapy: efficacy, toxicity, and immunologic effects of early gestation recombinant adenovirus. British Association of Paediatric Surgeons. J. Pediatr. Surg. **34:** 235–241.
70. TAJIMA, T. *et al.* 1999. Restoration of adrenal steroidogenesis by adenovirus-mediated transfer of human cytochromeP450 21-hydroxylase into the adrenal gland of 21-hydroxylase-deficient mice. Gene Ther. **6:** 1898–1903.
71. HANKE, C.J. *et al.* 2000. Inhibition of adrenal cell aldosterone synthesis by endogenous nitric oxide release. Hypertension **35:** 324–328.
72. CHUMAN, Y., Z. ZHAN & T. FOJO. 2000. Construction of gene therapy vectors targeting adrenocortical cells: enhancement of activity and specificity with agents modulating the cyclic adenosine 3′,5′-monophosphate pathway. J. Clin. Endocrinol. Metab. **85:** 253–262.
73. ALESCI, S. *et al.* 2002. Adenoviral vectors can impair adrenocortical steroidogenesis: clinical implications for natural infections and gene therapy. Proc. Natl. Acad. Sci. USA **99:** 7484–7489.
74. HORNSBY, P.J. 2001. Transplantation of adrenocortical cells. Rev. Endocr. Metab. Disord. **2:** 313–321.
75. LITTLEY, M.D. *et al.* 1991. Endocrine and reproductive dysfunction following fractionated total body irradiation in adults. Q. J. Med. **78:** 265–274.
76. DAVIS, J.R. *et al.* 1999. Gene therapy for pituitary tumours. Endocr. Relat. Cancer **6:** 475–481.
77. CASTRO, M.G. *et al.* 1999. Cell-type specific expression in the pituitary: physiology and gene therapy. Biochem. Soc. Trans. **27:** 858–863.
78. LEE, E.J. *et al.* 1999. Targeted expression of toxic genes directed by pituitary hormone promoters: a potential strategy for adenovirus-mediated gene therapy of pituitary tumors. J. Clin. Endocrinol. Metab. **84:** 786–794.
79. NEILL, J.D. *et al.* 1999. High efficiency method for gene transfer in normal pituitary gonadotropes: adenoviral-mediated expression of G protein-coupled receptor kinase 2 suppresses luteinizing hormone secretion. Endocrinology **140:** 2562–2569.
80. CASTRO, M.G. *et al.* 1997. Expression of transgenes in normal and neoplastic anterior pituitary cells using recombinant adenoviruses: long term expression, cell cycle dependency, and effects on hormone secretion. Endocrinology **138:** 2184–2194.
81. WINDEATT, S. *et al.* 2000. Adenovirus-mediated herpes simplex virus type-1 thymidine kinase gene therapy suppresses oestrogen-induced pituitary prolactinomas. J. Clin. Endocrinol. Metab. **85:** 1296–1305.
82. WOLF, D. *et al.* 1988. Retrovirus-mediated gene transfer of beta-nerve growth factor into mouse pituitary line AtT-20. Mol. Biol. Med. **5:** 43–59.
83. HORELLOU, P. *et al.* 1989. Retroviral transfer of a human tyrosine hydroxylase cDNA in various cell lines: regulated release of dopamine in mouse anterior pituitary AtT-20 cells. Proc. Natl. Acad. Sci. USA **86:** 7233–7237.
84. GOYA, R.G. *et al.* 1998. Use of recombinant herpes simplex virus type 1 vectors for gene transfer into tumour and normal anterior pituitary cells. Mol. Cell. Endocrinol. **139:** 199–207.

Index of Contributors

Alesci, S., 177–192

Bergström, M., 159–169
Bravo, E.L., 1–10
Brouwers, F.M., 11–28

Carrasquillo, J.A., 170–176
Charmandari, E., 101–111
Chen, C.C., 170–176
Chrousos, G.P., 101–111, 177–192

Eisenhofer, G., vii–viii, 29–40, 170–176
Eriksson, B., 159–169

Funder, J.W., 89–100

Goldstein, D.S., 170–176
Grossman, A., 119–133

Ilias, I., 134–144

Jackson, R.V., 77–88
Juhlin, C., 159–169

Kino, T., 101–111
Koch, C.A., 11–28

Lafferty, A., 77–88
Långström, B., 159–169
Lenders, J.W.M., 29–40
Morris, D., 119–133

Mullen, N., 134–144

New, M.I., 145–154
Newman, K.D., 155–158
Nieman, L.K., 112–118, 134–144

Öberg, K., 159–169
Örlefors, H., 159–169

Pacak, K., vii–viii, 11–28, 29–40, 170–176, 177–192
Ponsky, T., 155–158

Rocha, R., 89–100

Sisson, J.C., 54–60
Stratakis, C., 77–88
Sundin, A., 159–169

Torpy, D.J., 77–88, 134–144

Vortmeyer, A.O., 11–28
Vottero, A., 101–111

Walther, M.M., 41–53
Whatley, M., 170–176

Young, W.F., Jr., 61–76

Zhuang, Z., 11–28

OHIO UNIVERSITY LIBRARY

Please return this book as soon as you have finished with it. In order to avoid a fine it must be returned by the latest date stamped below. All books are subject to recall after two weeks or immediately if needed for reserve.

CF